Table of

Table of Contents

Introduction

About the Author

Chapter 1 - The Cycle

Chapter 2 - PMS & Cravings

Chapter 3 - The Pill

Chapter 4 - Hypothalamic Amenorrhea (HA)

Chapter 5 - PCOS

Chapter 6 - Endometriosis

Chapter 7 - Pre & Post Natal

Chapter 8 - Perimenopause and Menopause

Chapter 9 - Thyroid

Chapter 10 - Your Cycles Leaves Clues

Conclusion

References

Introduction

Before I go into this book.

This book is not meant for medical advice. The main aim is to educate women at all stages of their lives and educate PT's, Nutritionists and partners along the way.

Over 51% of the world are women and none of us would be here if the cycle wasn't present. Yes, your mom has/had a cycle at some stage of their lives.

A lot of change happens for women from puberty, to your first cycle, to trying to conceive, to perimenopause to menopause. All of these have different difficulties and it can bring with it an array of challenges but you are not alone.

The purpose of this book is to make sure the next generation of women talk about their bodies and celebrate their uniqueness. Yes, you are all unique.

Embrace your individuality and own it.

Some of the topics that I cover in this book include:

- Your cycle
- Training & Nutrition around your cycle
- Pre and Post Natal Training and Nutrition
- PMS
- Perimenopause & Menopause
- PCOS
- Endometriosis
- Amenorrhea

There is so much in this book and if you are reading this, thank you!

If you learn even one thing then please share and spread the word.

About the Author

Shane is the Director of Shane Walsh Fitness, an online coaching service that has worked with nearly a thousand women to help them to understand their body and provide them with the body confidence they have always wanted.

Shane provides education to clients on all areas of Female Health, including PCOS, Perimenopause, Menopause, Endometriosis, Pre and Post Natal Training and Nutrition, Contraception, HA and how to manage cravings and PMS.

Shane is a fully qualified Nutritionist, Personal trainer and is Certified in Pre and Post Natal Exercise from NTC.

Shane is the host of the Shane Walsh Podcast which is one of the top Nutrition Podcasts on Apple in Ireland. The podcast is available to download on iTunes and Spotify.

Some of the guests that Shane has had include the likes of Lara Briden, Dr. Stacy Sims, Aisling O'Kelly, Diren Kartal, Siobhan O'Hagan, Sinead Hegarty, Clare Goodwin, Jay Alderton to name but a few.

The purpose of this Book is to get rid of the stigma attached to women and to help educate women to understand their body and get rid of the charlatans that are currently in the industry.

Chapter 1 - The Cycle

Before we go into this chapter and the book itself the most important statement in the book is the next line.

"Every woman is unique, every woman has different feelings, symptoms, length of cycles are different. Embrace your uniqueness as being the same as everyone is boring".

If you can understand how your body works for you after reading this book and in particular this chapter then it's a massive win. If you understand your body for you, it provides you with the freedom to make your body work for you not the other way around.

So, let's get started with understanding the basics of the cycle.

From working with nearly a thousand women (at the time of writing this) it is so important to realise that you are all different. Not everyone's symptoms will be the same. Some women may get more severe symptoms than others and others may feel no symptoms at all.

It's also important to note that Ovulation doesn't happen every month for every woman.

Some conditions may interfere with ovulation, such as endometriosis and PCOS (Polycystic Ovarian Syndrome), make sure to check out the chapters on these conditions in more detail later in the book. If you are not getting a monthly period, please talk to your doctor.

Before we go into more detail, we need to start with the basics and understand what happens to your body during the course of a month.

Each month during the years between puberty and menopause, a woman's body goes through a number of changes to get it ready for a possible pregnancy. This series of hormone-driven events is called the menstrual cycle.

The menstrual cycle, which is counted from the first day of one period to the first day of the next, isn't the same for every woman. Menstrual flow might occur every 21 to 35 days and last two to seven days.

During each menstrual cycle, an egg develops and is released from the ovaries. The lining of the uterus builds up. If a pregnancy doesn't happen, the uterine lining sheds during a menstrual period. Then the cycle starts again.

The menstrual cycle is more than just the period. In fact, the period is just the first phase of the cycle. The menstrual cycle is actually made up of two cycles that interact and overlap—one happening in the ovaries and one in the uterus. The brain, ovaries, and uterus work together and communicate through hormones (chemical signals sent through the blood from one part of the body to another) to keep the cycle going.

A woman's menstrual cycle is divided into four

phases:

- menstrual phase
- follicular phase
- ovulation phase
- luteal phase

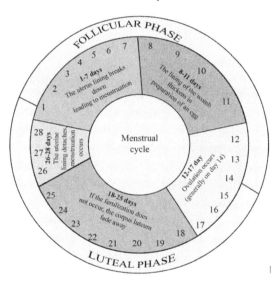

The length of each phase can differ from woman to woman, and it can change over time. This is where embracing your uniqueness can be empowering and provide you with the freedom of understanding how your body works once and for all.

Your menstrual cycle might be regular — about the same length every month — or somewhat irregular, and your period might be light or heavy, painful or pain-free, long or short, and still be considered normal. Within a broad range, "normal" is what's normal for you.

If it becomes irregular for either short or long there is normally a reason for this and it is important to be in tune with how your body works for you. This is where tracking your cycle comes into play.

Keep in mind that use of certain types of contraception, such as extended-cycle birth control pills and intrauterine devices (IUDs), will alter your menstrual cycle. Talk to your health care provider about what to expect. (Please see the chapter on Contraception later in the book)

At what age does the cycle start and finish?

Girls start menstruating at the average age of 12. However, girls can begin menstruating as early as 8 years of age or as late as 16 years of age.

When you get close to menopause things change. The Menopause chapter goes into things in more detail so please read that chapter.

Women stop menstruating at menopause. The average age for menopause to start in the UK is currently 51. At menopause, a woman stops producing eggs (stops ovulating). Menopause is defined as one year without periods, and after this time a woman can no longer become pregnant (check out the chapter on menopause).

What happens at each stage?

Menstrual phase

The menstrual phase is the first stage of the menstrual cycle. It's also when you get your period.

This phase starts when an egg from the previous cycle isn't fertilized. Because pregnancy hasn't taken place, levels of the hormones estrogen and progesterone drop.

The thickened lining of your uterus, which would support a pregnancy, is no longer needed, so it sheds through your vagina. During your period, you release a combination of blood, mucus, and tissue from your uterus.

You may have period symptoms that include:
- cramps
- tender breasts
- bloating
- mood swings
- irritability
- headaches
- tiredness
- low back pain

On average, women are in the menstrual phase of their cycle for 3 to 7 days. Some women have longer periods than others.

Follicular phase

The follicular phase starts on the first day of your period (so there is some overlap with the menstrual phase) and ends when you ovulate. Think of it this way: the Follicular phase = increasing estrogen.

It starts when the hypothalamus (The hypothalamus is a part of the brain that has a vital role in controlling many bodily functions including the release of hormones from the pituitary gland) sends a signal to your pituitary gland to release follicle-stimulating hormone (FSH). This hormone stimulates your ovaries to produce around 5 to 20 small sacs called follicles. Each follicle contains an immature egg.

Only the healthiest egg will eventually mature. (On rare occasions, a woman may have two eggs mature.) The rest of the follicles will be reabsorbed into your body.

The maturing follicle sets off a surge in estrogen that thickens the lining of your uterus. This creates a nutrient-rich environment for an embryo to grow.

The average follicular phase lasts for about 16 days. It can range from 11 to 27 days, depending on your cycle. The length of your follicular phase depends in part on the amount of time it takes one dominant follicle to emerge. When the follicle is slow to mature, this phase will last longer. Your whole menstrual cycle will also be longer as a result.

A long follicular phase means that it takes more time for your body to ovulate. Using birth control pills for a long time can lengthen your follicular phase. Low vitamin D levels have also been linked to a longer follicular phase.

Women with a long follicular phase are just as likely to get pregnant as those with a statistically more normal follicular phase. Having a longer cycle shouldn't affect your fertility.

Having a short follicular phase could impact your likelihood of conceiving, though. It may be a sign that your ovaries are aging and you're getting closer to menopause.

The follicular phase may start to get shorter when you're in your late 30s, even if you still get a monthly period. Hormone levels change during this time. Your FSH levels still rise, but your LH levels stay low. This causes a follicle to ripen too quickly. The egg inside that follicle may not be mature enough or ready to fertilize. This makes pregnancy more unlikely.

During the follicular phase of the cycle—from the start of your period until ovulation—estrogen levels are high. You may notice some changes throughout your body, some of these may include, one of these being before ovulation, you may notice that their skin and hair are less oily (though we don't know for sure that the increase in estrogen causes these changes).

Another element to be aware of is that your cervical fluid changes throughout the follicular phase:

- *Early-to mid follicular*: dry/sticky
- *Mid-to-late follicular:* thick/sticky/creamy
- *Late follicular to ovulation*: wet and slippery, like an egg white

- Some people notice an increase in their sex drive around ovulation

One of other major things to note is that your body temperature may change during this phase. Tracking your basal body temperature can help you figure out on which days of the month you'll have the best odds of conceiving. Your basal body temperature is your lowest temperature when you're at rest.

To measure basal body temperature, keep a thermometer at your bedside and take your temperature upon waking, before you even get out of bed. This should be done at the same time each morning.

In the follicular phase of your cycle, your basal body temperature should be between 97.0 and 97.5°F (36°C). When you ovulate, your temperature will rise and remain higher during the luteal phase, confirming that the follicular phase is over.

Ovulation phase

Rising estrogen levels during the follicular phase trigger your pituitary gland to release luteinizing hormone (LH). This is what starts the process of ovulation.

Ovulation is when your ovary releases a mature egg. The egg travels down the fallopian tube toward the uterus to be fertilized by sperm.

The ovulation phase is the only time during your

menstrual cycle when you can get pregnant. You can tell that you're ovulating by symptoms like these:

- a slight rise in basal body temperature (normally 0.4 degrees Celsius)
- thicker discharge that has the texture of egg whites

Ovulation happens at around day 14 if you have a 28-day cycle — right in the middle of your menstrual cycle. It lasts about 24 hours. After a day, the egg will die or dissolve if it isn't fertilized.

When you want to have a baby, you can improve your chance of getting pregnant if you know about ovulation and the 'fertile window' in the menstrual cycle. This is the time of the month when you're most likely to get pregnant. If you are trying to have a baby outside of the window you may as well be using a branch of a tree, you won't get pregnant.

Check out the section later in the book on fertility and how you can improve this

Luteal phase

Think of the Follicular phase as lower estrogen. After the follicle releases its egg, it changes into the corpus luteum. This structure releases hormones, mainly progesterone and some estrogen. The rise in hormones keeps your uterine lining thick and ready for a fertilized egg to implant.

If you do get pregnant, your body will produce

human chorionic gonadotropin (hCG). This is the hormone pregnancy tests detect. It helps maintain the corpus luteum and keeps the uterine lining thick.

If you don't get pregnant, the corpus luteum will shrink away and be resorbed. This leads to decreased levels of estrogen and progesterone (calming hormone), which causes the onset of your period. The uterine lining will shed during your period.

During this phase, if you don't get pregnant, you may experience symptoms of premenstrual syndrome (PMS). These include:

- bloating
- breast swelling, pain, or tenderness
- mood changes
- headache
- weight gain
- changes in sexual desire
- food cravings
- trouble sleeping
- The luteal phase lasts for 11 to 17 days.
- The average length is 14 days.

Please check out the next chapter on how to manage PMS and how to manage the various symptoms that may appear.

Identifying common issues

Every woman's menstrual cycle is different. Some women get their period at the same time each month. Others are more irregular. Some women bleed more heavily or for a longer number of days than others.

Your menstrual cycle can also change during certain times of your life. For example, it can get more irregular as you get close to menopause.

One way to find out if you're having any issues with your menstrual cycle is to track your periods. Write down when they start and end. Also record any changes to the amount or number of days you bleed, and whether you have spotting between periods (see later on the chapter on the importance of tracking your cycle).

A number of things can alter your menstrual cycle so it is very important to understand what you are putting into your body, what your body is going through and check in with your doctor if you feel something isn't right.

- *Birth control.* The birth control pill may make your periods shorter and lighter. While on some pills, you won't get a period at all. Remember birth control stops you from ovulating.
- *Pregnancy.* Your periods should stop during pregnancy. Missed periods are one of the most obvious first signs that you're pregnant.

- *Polycystic ovary syndrome (PCOS).* This hormonal imbalance prevents an egg from developing normally in the ovaries. PCOS causes irregular menstrual cycles and missed periods.
- *Uterine fibroids.* These noncancerous growths in your uterus can make your periods longer and heavier than usual.
- *Eating disorders.* Anorexia, bulimia, and other eating disorders can disrupt your menstrual cycle and make your periods stop.
- *Pelvic inflammatory disease (PID).* This infection of the reproductive organs can cause irregular menstrual bleeding.

What can you do to prevent menstrual irregularities?

For some women, use of birth control pills (see chapter on birth control for more information) can help regulate menstrual cycles. If you are relying on the pill to regulate your cycle and you come off it, the cycle may remain irregular like it was before you started taking the pill. It's like sticking a band aid over a broken arm.

In addition, consult your healthcare provider if:

- Your periods suddenly stop for more than 90 days — and you're not pregnant
- Your periods become erratic after having been regular
- You bleed for more than seven days

- You bleed more heavily than usual or soak through more than one pad or tampon every hour or two
- Your periods are less than 21 days or more than 35 days apart
- You bleed between periods
- You develop severe pain during your period
- You suddenly get a fever and feel sick after using tampons

If you have questions or concerns about your menstrual cycle, talk to your health care provider.

Every woman's menstrual cycle is different. What's normal for you might not be normal for someone else.

It's important to get familiar with your cycle and that's where tracking your cycle can really help.

Importance of tracking your cycle

Understanding your period can tell you more about yourself than you might imagine. I may repeat myself a lot in this book about the importance of tracking your cycle and symptoms and that's because I have seen this first hand with clients how it can change someone's life.

It can help you understand your unique patterns.

The simplest way to track your cycle is to log when your period occurs so you can start to understand your average cycle length. Everybody is different, and having an unpredictable period is more common than you think. A 28-35 day cycle is a global average, but may not be your personal average. If you are aware of your cycle, you will naturally feel more in control–and less likely to be surprised by your next period.

You'll know when you ovulate

There are common misconceptions about how pregnancy occurs: that you can only get pregnant on your day of ovulation, or that you can get pregnant all the time. Neither of these are true. During the days leading up to and after ovulation, pregnancy is possible. Tracking ovulation through the apps or methods I list below can really help alongside measuring your body temperature.

It will increase your awareness of your overall health and wellness

Your menstrual cycle is a direct indicator of your overall health, and periods are your body's way of telling you that things are working as they should. Having an extremely unpredictable or heavy period, or skipping a period, can indicate an existing underlying condition. By tracking and logging various details of your cycle, you will be able to recall things that you might otherwise forget when speaking with your healthcare provider.

It can tell you a lot about your individual sex drive

Tracking your sex drive and sexual activity can help determine patterns in your cycle. Around ovulation, you might notice spikes in your sexual desire. Sex is healthy, so being aware of your sexual activity by tracking in a fun way to know when you might feel the most desire (or not).

You can understand and manage your mood

It's not just about PMS. Hormonal changes throughout the menstrual cycle have been suggested to cause changes in mood like irritability, anxiety, or feeling more affectionate. Learning when these changes happen can be another piece of information to help understand the rhythm of your cycle.

You can understand when you are stronger in the gym

Yes, the cycle has an impact on your strength, energy and ability for certain types of exercise. This is discussed later on in this chapter in a lot more detail. This could be the difference between you getting Personal Bests in the gym or running yourself into the ground with more HIIT style training.

The best methods of tracking your cycle include:

- Apps like Kindara
- Clue
- Natural cycles
- And a good old-fashioned pen and paper

Knowing your body can save you a lot of frustration and a lot of heart ache so if you are not tracking download an app and get tracking today.

What about if you are on the pill?

You do NOT get a real period when on the contraceptive pill.

Unlike the combined pill, the copper coil does not stop ovulation, so you will still have a "real period" and ovulate.

The bleeding you get when you're on the pill is not the same as a menstrual period.

Your period on the pill is technically called withdrawal bleeding, referring to the withdrawal of hormones in your pill, and in your body. The drop in hormone levels causes the lining of your uterus (the endometrium) to shed. This bleeding may be slightly different than the period you had before taking the pill. It also may change over time while taking the pill.

Should you ovulate while on the pill?

If you take your pill consistently and correctly, you shouldn't ovulate. This is the primary way the pill prevents pregnancy. In a usual (no-pill) cycle, the body's natural reproductive hormones fluctuate up and down, taking your body through a process of preparing an egg for release, releasing that egg, and preparing your uterus to accept a potentially fertilized egg.

The hormones in the contraceptive pill stop and prevent your ovaries from preparing and releasing eggs. They stop the usual hormonal "cycling", including ovulation, the typical growth of the endometrium, and the natural period.

There is a full chapter on the pill and the benefits and disadvantages of each one so please head to that chapter for more information. If you are someone who is on the pill your PMS symptoms may change slightly as will your energy at a certain time of the month for training. Please keep a log of your symptoms.

What if you don't have a cycle?

Your cycle is key. If you don't have a cycle there is a reason for it and it is so important that you investigate it. If you don't have a cycle, it may be something called Hypothalamic Amenorrhea. Hypothalamic Amenorrhea is defined as the lack of a menstrual cycle period of more than six months when no medical diagnosis can be found. The last part of this sentence is very important.

The no medical diagnosis means your doctor should have ruled out other conditions such as thyroid disease, celiac disease, PCOS, high prolactin and others.

Think of your cycle like the cog that keeps your body functioning. It is a powerful tool and if it's not working properly then something is not right and the body is not at optimal health and is trying to provide you with feedback that something is not quite right.

Another element that could be at play is if you are someone who has been taking the pill for years and has decided to come off it for personal reasons. It can take up to 6 months for hormones to sync back up but please link in with your GP and ask questions if you are uncertain of anything.

Please go to the Hypothalamic Amenorrhea chapter for full details on this.

The next section is going to talk about how you should train or train your clients at certain stages of your cycle. This is game changing information for so many.

How should you train around your cycle?

There is more and more research going into how women should train around their cycles. For a very long time the research on training was mainly done on men and as we should know men are completely different. There is an amazing quote from Dr.Stacy Sims that sums this up brilliantly "women are not small men". More research is being conducted and needs to be conducted in order to get a better picture. What is said now could be outdated in a couple of years.

Scientific studies are also exploring how fluctuations of hormones across the menstrual cycle can lead to different outcomes in training.

Tracking your cycle will play a massive role in how you should train so if you still haven't loaded the apps please do so now.

Here are some tips with your cycle in mind:

Don't skip strength training in the first part of your cycle

Several studies have looked at differences in responses to strength training in the follicular phase (the time from your period until ovulation), versus training in the luteal phase (from ovulation until your period).

Some research has found that strength training during the follicular phase resulted in higher increases in muscle strength compared to training in the luteal phase.

If you start paying attention to your cycle phases, you may find your strength training pays off the most in your follicular phase.

In plain English: NEVER skip leg day before you ovulate!

Watch out for tendon injuries on fertile days

A startling statistic for people playing sports is that women are 3 to 6 times more likely than men to have injuries to the anterior cruciate ligament (ACL).

A recent meta-review of studies looked at how hormonal changes may impact tendon laxity and risk of tendon injury. It found the risk was highest in the days leading up to ovulation, when estrogen is high. The luteal phase was associated with the lowest risk. More research is needed, but it's worth doing longer warm-up exercises and not overstretching during your potential fertile days.

Don't beat yourself up in the second part of your cycle

In the second part of your cycle, progesterone rises significantly. Your body temperature is also higher during this phase—body temp shoots up by at least 0.4 degrees Celsius after ovulation and stays high until menstruation. Your body is preparing for a potential pregnancy, should an egg have been fertilized at ovulation.

As a result, you may find that you don't have as much endurance during your luteal phase. You may not be able to hit max lifts, and may feel worse in training compared to the first part of your cycle.

So, don't judge the results of your training based on your performance in this phase alone. Decreased performance is a perfectly normal experience in the luteal phase of your cycle.

For example, training sessions feel much more challenging in this period. To give an example from a few weeks ago: one of my clients was trying to do 3x3 front squats at 90 percent of her 1 rep max, yet she could barely eke out the reps at 85 percent. She was wondering how she ever lifted at 90 percent!

Take rest days in the second part of your cycle

Based on the info above, you might want to schedule your rest days during your luteal phase.

That doesn't mean you should entirely skip training in this phase, as you'll still improve from strength training in the luteal phase. If you're not sure exactly when you're ovulating, or you want a baseline for how long your average luteal phase tends to be, try taking ovulation tests for a few cycles (ovulation can shift cycle-to-cycle, but it's usually your follicular phase that's getting shorter or longer).

Also, if you want to take time off from training for vacation, your luteal phase is a great time to take it in order to reduce impact on your strength goals. These are very rough guidelines and I have seen other women feel stronger the week before and feel flattened around ovulation. When you notice a trend of when you feel more fatigued, please note that this is not the time to do loads of extra cardio or HIIT style workouts. Sometimes your body needs you to think of it like a phone and recharge it.

Don't be hard on yourself if your workouts aren't as good at certain times of the month. It's normal. Hormones are chemical messengers in your body. Just like melatonin signals us when it's time to sleep, different hormone levels may signal when it's time for our body to hit the gym or take it easy.

Keep in mind that everyone is different; just because hormonal fluctuations make you feel like you should want to train hard during the follicular phase or take it easy during the luteal phase, this doesn't mean you need to do that. A good training approach for you is one that makes you feel good!

Lastly, be sure to consult with your doctor or health

practitioner if you have any concerns regarding your menstrual cycle and training.

Nutrition around your cycle

Adjusting your diet to support your fluctuating hormones can be a game changer when it comes to taking charge of your own health, but it's especially helpful if you struggle with PMS, painful periods or other symptoms of hormonal imbalance.

The reason?

All the hormones in your endocrine system that work together to carry out vital functions and promote homeostasis (the state of equilibrium) in the body, are influenced by many factors, including what you eat.

In particular the balance of progesterone and estrogen (the primary cycle hormones that fluctuate throughout our monthly cycles) is imperative not only for hormone health, but overall physical mental and emotional well-being.

Keeping your blood sugar levels steady also contributes to overall hormone balance, helping to reduce mood swings and better manage weight, sleep and cravings (check out the next chapter for advice on managing cravings).

To do this, try eating balanced meals filled with fibre and protein at regular intervals, and being mindful of the types of sugars and carbohydrates that we are eating.

Please note that every woman is different and it is so important to understand your body.

How to fuel yourself at each stage of the cycle?

What to eat during Menstruation?

Because of this hormonal dip, energy levels are likely to be low, so support the body with plenty of water and unprocessed, nutrient rich foods that keep energy and blood sugar levels steady. A good mix of lean proteins, healthy fats and low GI complex carbohydrates such as root vegetables, wholegrain and legumes, can support the energy-intensive process of menstruation.

Include plenty of iron-rich foods such as lentils, kelp, pumpkin seeds, dried prunes and spinach and, if you eat animal products, beef, eggs and fish are also a good source of iron. This is also a timely moment to make decent food choices as lower levels of hormones may make it a time of the month when women often report feeling less hungry. Smoothies are a great choice around this time if you are not hungry.

Some women have also reported increased hunger during this phase so that is why it is so important to understand your body. If you are counting calories or dieting now is not the time to be doing so.

If you are dieting, research would encourage you to increase calories by 200-300 (woman dependant).

For example, if you are on 1,600 calories per day. Then increase your calorie intake to 1,800 - 1,900 calories per day. (These calories are not tailored to anyone and is for this example only)

What to eat during the Follicular Phase?

Hormone levels, while still low, are beginning to rise as your egg follicles mature, in preparation for ovulation.

You may be starting to feel more energised, and potentially including more exercise, so this is a good time to incorporate light, fresh and vibrant foods, such as salads and fermented foods like kefir, probiotic yoghurt or sauerkraut, which support gut health and detoxification.

With rising estrogen, some women find that they have more energy, focus and willpower at this time.

What to eat during the Ovulation Phase?

Once the egg has matured, we move into the ovulatory phase. Hormone levels are rising, particularly estrogen as it aids in the ovulation process.

Your basal body temperature also increases, which can impact increased energy levels. Excess estrogen can have a negative impact on our cycle including breast tenderness and increased spots, so nutrients that support the liver to remove estrogen are good.

Foods like Quinoa, Eggs, Kale, Radishes, Whole Grain options like breads, pasta, rice and also include fruits like berries, citrus and papaya can help you around this time of the month.

Without energy in your body ovulation cannot not occur so it is essential that you fill up your body. Carbs will be the key that starts the engine so please do not fear them they are essential for your bodies overall health.

What to eat during the Luteal Phase?

Hormone levels reach their peak as you approach menstruation and many women experience PMS around this time.

It is possible to help manage pre-period moods and discomforts through food choices: if you experience water retention in the form of swollen breasts and bloating, reduce foods high in salt as they can exacerbate the problem, due to salt's anti-diuretic effects on the body.

The same applies to sugar; if you are prone to cravings, they may be at their highest during this week and carbohydrates may be what you are craving, however just ensure they are complex ones such as like brown rice, pasta or bread (the husks are filled with energy with and stress- supporting B vitamins and fibre to help curb cravings and balance those moods). It is important that you read the next chapter on the truth of sugar cravings.

This is also a good time of the month to cut down on

caffeine and alcohol, as these stimulants can aggravate PMS- triggered anxiety and mood shifts.

Coffee and alcohol can also interfere with the absorption of essential vitamins and minerals required for optimal menstrual health, so try some alternatives like sparkling fruit water, herbal teas, chicory root or swap your morning latte for a caffeine free one.

At this time of the month research would encourage women to increase their calories by roughly 200-300 calories in order to help with cravings. For example, if you are currently eating 1,600 calories per day, then increase your calories to 1,800 - 1,900 per day. This will be a game changer.

Sounds like a lot of planning?

Don't sweat it. Aim to make small changes and keep a note of what works for you.

If you have PCOS, Endometriosis or Amenorrhea please reach out to your GP, Dietitian, Nutritionist to lead you in the right direction. These are all manageable with the right direction. Please see the chapters on these topics later in the book for more information.

Remember you only have one body so it's important to use it to the best of its ability.

You got this.

Digestion and the Menstrual Cycle

<u>The importance of digestion on your cycle</u>

"No gut health, no happy hormones."

The point is that your gut health has an impact on your hormones, your menstrual cycle, and even any PMS symptoms you may experience.

We need to start with the basics first before we go any further

<u>What is the microbiome?</u>

The microbiome may sound like an exhibition at Epcot, but it's actually one of the most important functioning areas of your body. Basically, your body is filled with tons of bacteria, viruses, and other tiny microorganisms naked to the human eye. They mostly live in your large intestine or on your skin, and they live in a little pocket within your large intestine. Those microbes in your intestines are what's known as your microbiome, and it's what we're referring to any time we say "gut health."

And it's totally normal and healthy to have these trillion (yes, trillion with a "t") bacteria, fungi, and viruses living in your body. In fact, you need them so your body can function, and you want a diverse microbiome because it's better for your health. The food you eat has a lot of impact on the diversity of your microbiome, but your microbiome can be impacted by lots of other factors.

How does your gut health impact your hormones?

On the highest level, an imbalanced microbiome has been correlated with hormonal imbalances—and on the flip side, having too much estrogen in your body can cause gut-related issues like bloating and fluid retention.

Here's a little more detail. When your ovaries make estrogen, the hormone then travels through your bloodstream before settling down in your liver. There, the estrogen is deactivated and sent to your intestine where the microbes live. Then, it's broken down by an enzyme so it can exit the body. But if that microbiome isn't functioning well, the estrogen will recirculate back through your body—and that could cause a hormonal imbalance.

How does your gut health impact your period?

So, if estrogen re-circulates through your body and you develop excess levels of it, you'll probably experience symptoms pretty similar to PMS: heavier periods, bloating, mood swings, and more.

So basically, the only way to get rid of your old estrogen is to go to the bathroom for a number 2. If you are looking to improve this, think fibre, fruit, veggies and water. Think of your cycle like a snake skin. It regenerates each month it needs to regenerate for a new cycle to emerge.

Fluctuating estrogen levels can impact the digestive tract, too, by leading to spasms in your intestines that can potentially cause diarrhea. Or, you could have the opposite issue and experience constipation due to a dip in estrogen, which slows digestion.

How do you take care of your gut health?

There are a few things you can do to care for your microbiome and your reproductive health. First, up your water intake and make sure you're eating a diet high in fibre; that'll help facilitate healthy digestion and stave off any diarrhoea or constipation.

Make sure you're paying attention to your stress levels. Psychological stress and sleep deprivation can upset the microbiome, so make sure you're exercising regularly, meditating, getting outside, or practicing any other self-care that you've found effective.

Finally, think about the variety of fruit and veggies. The amount of fibre that someone should consume in a day varies from 20-35g per day (depending on where you get your research and depending on your gender). So rather than trying to aim for another target, why not aim to get veggies and fruit into most of your meals. A great hack is using the likes of flax seeds and chia seeds. They are cheap and cheerful too!

A lot of what can be managed with the gut involves managing stress, lifestyle, alcohol intake, water intake and sleep.

If you are struggling to go to the bathroom, up that fibre.

What about losing weight?

<u>Compare your like weeks with your like weeks</u>

"Why does my weight go up in a certain week?"

This is one of the most common questions I hear as a Nutritionist.

During your period, it's normal to gain three to five pounds that goes away after a few days of bleeding. It's a physical symptom of premenstrual syndrome (PMS). I have even had some clients gain up to 12 lbs during certain stages of their cycles.

Weight gain and that bloated, sore feeling in your abdomen are common symptoms during your period. You might feel this way for a number of reasons.

Hormonal changes

Hormonal changes can cause weight gain by increasing water retention.

In the days before your period, estrogen and progesterone rapidly decrease. This tells your body that it's time to begin menstruation.

Estrogen and progesterone also control the way your body regulates fluid. When these hormones fluctuate, the tissues in your body accumulate more water. The result is water retention.

Water retention

Water retention may cause swelling or puffiness in your breasts, stomach, or extremities. This increases body weight, but not fat.

Water retention is a common PMS symptom. It affects 92 percent of women who menstruate, so you are not alone!

Bloating

Period bloating or stomach cramps can make your clothes feel tight and uncomfortable. This isn't true weight gain, but you might feel like you've gained a few extra pounds.

During your period, hormonal changes can increase gas in your gastrointestinal (GI) tract and cause bloating. Water retention in your abdomen may also lead to bloating.

Bloating can be described as feeling tight or swollen in your stomach or other parts of your body.

Stomach cramps

Stomach cramps can also cause the sensation of weight gain. These cramps are caused by chemicals called prostaglandins that are released by your uterus. Prostaglandins make your uterus contract and shed its lining. This causes abdominal pain during your period.

Bloating may start five days before your period and continue into the first few days of menstruation. Stomach cramps, which begin one or two days before your period, can also last for a few days.

My #1 tip here for my clients is compare your like weeks with your like weeks.

What do I mean by this?

Compare the week of your cycle in October to the week of your cycle in November, week after your cycle in October to week after your cycle in November and so on. This will allow you to notice a trend over time. It is not your fault that your weight goes up. In fact, it is a normal thing to happen and it is something that if you are staying honest and staying consistent then it will be what you do over time that will make the difference.

Please be aware that the weight increase is not fat gain.

Think averages not fluctuations.

If you are someone who struggles with the weighing scales, I would highly recommend to stay off it more than stepping on it. Focus on non-scale victories (NSV's) like how you feel in your clothes, your strength, your libido and your energy levels.

Conclusion

The cycle is something that should be celebrated as without it none of us would be here on this planet.

Some women may not feel like this through various symptoms and conditions but things can be managed through lifestyle and diet.

Remember that you are unique and to understand your body for you is the biggest thing you can do for you. If you don't understand how your body works how can you expect anyone else to.

The next chapter is on PMS and how to manage the various symptoms.

Remember the sentence "*women are not small men*".

Chapter 2 - PMS & Cravings

What is PMS?

Premenstrual syndrome (PMS) or premenstrual tension (PMT), which are the same thing, is a condition that affects a woman's emotions, physical health, and behavior during certain days of the menstrual cycle, generally just before her menses.

PMS is a very common condition. Its symptoms affect more than 90 percent of menstruating women.

PMS symptoms can start five to 11 days before menstruation and typically go away once menstruation begins. The cause of PMS is unknown.

However, many researchers believe that it's related to a change in both sex hormone and serotonin levels at the beginning of the menstrual cycle.

Serotonin levels affect mood. Serotonin is a chemical in your brain and gut that affects your moods, emotions, and thoughts.

Levels of estrogen and progesterone increase during certain times of the month. An increase in these hormones can cause mood swings, anxiety, and irritability. Ovarian steroids also modulate activity in parts of your brain associated with premenstrual symptoms.

Risk factors for premenstrual syndrome include:

- a history of depression or mood disorders, such as postpartum depression or bipolar disorder
- a family history of PMS
- a family history of depression
- domestic violence
- substance abuse
- physical trauma
- emotional trauma

Associated conditions include:
- dysmenorrhea
- major depressive disorder
- seasonal affective disorder
- generalized anxiety disorder
- schizophrenia

Symptoms of PMS

A woman's menstrual cycle can last on average between 28-35 days. As I have mentioned before it is essential that you track your cycle (use apps like Natural Cycles, Kindara, Clue or a good old-fashioned pen and paper) and this will enable you to pre-empt when you may be expecting cravings, lower mood or a drop in overall energy.

The symptoms of PMS are usually mild or moderate. Nearly 80 percent of women report one or more symptoms that do not substantially affect daily functioning, according to the journal American Family Physician.

Twenty to 32 percent of women report moderate to

severe symptoms that affect some aspect of life, while three to eight percent report PMDD. The severity of symptoms can vary by individual and by month.

The symptoms of PMS include:

- abdominal bloating
- abdominal pain
- sore breasts
- acne
- food cravings, especially for sweets
- constipation
- diarrhea
- headaches
- sensitivity to light or sound
- fatigue
- irritability
- changes in sleep patterns
- anxiety
- depression
- sadness
- emotional outbursts

PMDD or severe PMS

Severe PMS: premenstrual dysphoric disorder

As mentioned in the previous section there is a severe type of PMS and it is important to chat with your doctor for the right diagnosis and treatment.

Severe PMS symptoms are rare. A small percentage of women who have severe symptoms have premenstrual dysphoric disorder (PMDD). PMDD affects between 3 and 8 percent of women.

The symptoms of PMDD may include:

- depression
- thoughts of suicide
- panic attacks
- extreme anxiety
- anger with severe mood swings
- crying spells
- a lack of interest in daily activities
- insomnia
- trouble thinking or focusing
- binge eating
- painful cramping
- bloating

The symptoms of PMDD may occur due to changes in your estrogen and progesterone levels. A connection between low serotonin levels and PMDD also exists.

Your doctor may do the following to rule out other medical problems:

- a physical exam
- a gynecological exam
- a complete blood count
- a liver function test

They may also recommend a psychiatric evaluation. A personal or family history of major depression, substance abuse, trauma, or stress can trigger or worsen PMDD symptoms.

Treatment for PMDD varies. Your doctor may recommend:

- daily exercise
- vitamin supplements, such as calcium, magnesium, and vitamin B-6
- a caffeine-free diet
- individual or group counselling
- stress management classes
- drospirenone and ethinyl estradiol tablet (Yaz)

If your PMDD symptoms still do not improve, your doctor may give you a selective serotonin reuptake inhibitor (SSRI) antidepressant. This medication increases serotonin levels in your brain and has many roles in regulating brain chemistry that are not limited to depression.

Your doctor may also suggest cognitive behavioural therapy (CBT), which is a form of counseling that can help you understand your thoughts and feelings and change your behaviour accordingly.

You can't prevent PMS or PMDD, but the treatments outlined above can help reduce the severity and duration of your symptoms.

When to see your doctor

See your doctor if physical pain, mood swings, and other symptoms start to affect your daily life, or if your symptoms don't go away.

The diagnosis is made when you have more than

one recurrent symptom in the correct time frame that is severe enough to cause impairment and is absent between menses and ovulation. Your doctor must also rule out other causes, such as:

- anaemia
- endometriosis
- thyroid disease
- irritable bowel syndrome (IBS)
- chronic fatigue syndrome
- connective tissue or rheumatologic diseases

Your doctor may ask about any history of depression or mood disorders in your family to determine whether your symptoms are the result of PMS or another condition. Some conditions, such as IBS, hypothyroidism, and pregnancy, have symptoms similar to PMS.

Your doctor may do a thyroid hormone test (see the chapter on Thyroid for more detail on this) to ensure that your thyroid gland is working properly, a pregnancy test, and possibly a pelvic exam to check for any gynaecological problems.

Keeping a diary of your symptoms is another way to determine if you have PMS. Use a calendar to keep track of your symptoms and menstruation every month. If your symptoms start around the same time each month, PMS is a likely cause.

Easing the symptoms of PMS

You can't cure PMS, but you can take steps to ease your symptoms.

There's a lot of conflicting scientific data out there regarding premenstrual syndrome (PMS). The most important thing to know about PMS is that most people experience some premenstrual symptoms, but that doesn't mean all people who menstruate have clinical PMS.

The best way to work around PMS is to figure out your unique patterns and what solutions work best for relieving your symptoms.

There are many ways to manage PMS symptoms, and not all are medical, scientific, or evidence-based. From a hot bath to your favourite comfort food, you don't always need evidence to know what makes you feel better. But if you're wondering about evidence-based solutions to PMS symptoms, here are some tips:

Eat a well-balanced diet to curb PMS symptoms

Make sure you're nourishing your body and eating a diet that provides it with the nutrients you need to thrive. Some research suggests that diets with adequate amounts of calcium and vitamin D may reduce the risk of PMS. Diets high in thiamine (vitamin B1) and riboflavin (vitamin B2) might also reduce the risk of experiencing PMS. Riboflavin has been shown to reduce the intensity of migraines by up to 50%. (Please check out the section on managing migraines for more information)

Work out regularly to prevent PMS symptoms

Exercise is a crucial part of a balanced life. It's

important not to just exercise when you have symptoms, but keep an ongoing exercise routine. Regular exercise may help with premenstrual headache, breast swelling, nausea, constipation, diarrhoea, bloating, and vomiting. The form of exercise that will help when you are in more discomfort could include Yoga, meditation, Pilates, yoga, walking and even lighten the weights that you are lifting in the gym (tracking your cycle will help you on this and you will notice when strength is up and when it dips).

Reduce stress to fight PMS symptoms

The combination of stress and premenstrual syndrome might create a cycle of exacerbation. If mild to moderate anxiety or irritation is part of your PMS pattern, try calming your nerves with yoga, breathing exercises, or mindfulness-based stress reduction. Some types of therapy like cognitive behavioural therapy may help with premenstrual symptoms, but more research is needed. Supplements like Ashwagandha have shown to help manage stress-like symptoms, it is important to get to the root cause of your stress first, e.g., if you work mental hours at work, I would start looking at managing your boundaries.

Supplement with Magnesium

Magnesium deficiency can cause a slew of symptoms, like anxiety, depression, irritability, and muscle weakness. Taking a magnesium supplement (100mg per day) has been suggested to help relieve

PMS-related symptoms, like headaches, bloating, and irritability. Pairing a magnesium supplement with B6 may be even more beneficial than taking magnesium alone.

Don't blame every bad mood on PMS

You are not a robot. A natural part of being human is to go through varying emotions. Before associating mood swings with PMS, consider other important predictors of daily mood like overall health and well-being. Considering PMS is used to discredit women in business and government, it's important to examine what it really is and you talk about it.

Could PMS really be a magnification of an existing health or mental health condition?

Blaming any uncomfortable symptoms that occur during the premenstrual phase on PMS could mask an underlying health issue. Anxiety and depression often get misdiagnosed as PMS. Other health conditions could also be misdiagnosed as PMS.

Look into taking Vitex

Other names for Vitex include Chaste Berry and Agnus Castus. Researchers believe that Vitex works by decreasing levels of the hormone prolactin. This helps rebalance other hormones, including estrogen and progesterone — thus reducing PMS symptoms.

In one study, women with PMS took Vitex agnus-castus during three consecutive menstrual cycles. In total, 93 percent of those given vitex reported a decrease in PMS symptoms, including:

- depression
- anxiety
- cravings

In two smaller studies, women with PMS were given 20 mg of Vitex agnus-castus per day or a placebo for three menstrual cycles. Twice as many women in the vitex group reported a decrease in symptoms including irritability, mood swings, headaches and breast fullness, compared to those given the placebo.

Vitex agnus-castus also appears to help reduce cyclic mastalgia, a type of breast pain linked to menstruation. Research suggests that it may be as effective as common drug treatment — but with far fewer side effects.

However, two recent reviews report that although vitex appears helpful in reducing PMS symptoms, its benefits may be overestimated. Better-designed studies may be needed before strong conclusions can be made. Whether it is a placebo effect or not it could be of benefit trying Vitex to help manage cravings.

Researchers report that 30–40 mg of dried fruit extracts, 3–6 grams of dried herb, or 1 gram of dried fruit per day appear safe.

Please do not take it if you are pregnant or breastfeeding or you are on medication for mental health.

Sleep & Fatigue management

Fatigue is one of the most common PMS symptoms. So, although it can be inconvenient and annoying to feel zapped of energy shortly before your period, it's completely normal.

In most cases, feeling tired before your period is nothing to be worried about. However, severe tiredness accompanied by certain emotions can be a sign of premenstrual dysphoric disorder (PMDD), a more severe form of PMS that often requires treatment.

Some studies have shown that 30% of women may have disrupted sleep patterns around ovulation time and even into the week after. Keep a log of your sleep pattern at certain times of the month and this will help you manage your sleep much better.

Your fatigue may also be caused by sleep issues linked to your physical premenstrual symptoms. PMS symptoms like bloating, cramping, and headaches can keep you up at night. Also, your body temperature tends to increase before your period, which can also make it more difficult to sleep.

If we as humans do not get enough sleep (7 to 9 hours is normally the recommended amount) we will notice a drop in energy. When our body has a drop in energy our brain will kick in and look for the quickest form of energy for the body and this where foods like processed foods, foods higher in carbs and sugar may come into the picture as they will provide us with a spike in energy. The spike in energy will be quickly followed by a drop and that vicious cycle will continue.

This is mainly due to the fact that when we get tired our hunger hormone goes into overdrive and our fullness hormone down regulates, leading to feeling hungrier more often. This is where those pesky cravings can really kick in (see later in the chapter on how to manage these cravings):

Some of the tools I work with client to manage their sleep include:

- *Create a healthy bedtime routine* - This is especially important in the days leading up to your period. A healthy bedtime routine can include taking a relaxing bath in the evening, skipping screen time at least an hour before bed, going to bed at the same time each night, and avoiding heavy meals and caffeine four to six hours before bed.
- *Try some carbs* (wholegrain if possible) before bed and this can help to increase the chances of getting better sleep.
- Eating a healthy diet and avoiding alcohol can help keep your energy levels up.
- *Prioritize your workout* - According to a 2015 Study, a moderate amount of aerobic exercise can help boost your energy levels, improve concentration, and ease most PMS symptoms. Try not to exercise within a

couple of hours of your bedtime as that may make it harder to fall asleep.
- *Keep your bedroom cool* - Use fans, an air conditioner, or open a window to keep your bedroom between 60 and 67°F (15.5 to 19.4°C). Doing so may help you fall asleep and stay asleep, despite your elevated body temperature.
- *Stay hydrated* - Don't forget to keep yourself hydrated by drinking at least 8 glasses of water each day. Being dehydrated can make you feel tired and lethargic, and may also make other PMS symptoms worse.
- *Try relaxation techniques* - Try using relaxation techniques that promote restfulness before bed. Some options include deep breathing exercises, meditation, and progressive relaxation therapy. You may also want to consider journaling or talk therapy to help unload extra stress you may feel before your period.

Alcohol

Having analysed 19 previously published studies of alcohol and PMS, researchers have found that the risk for PMS risk was 45% higher in women who reported drinking than in non-drinkers. Women who were heavy drinkers, (drinking more than one drink per day) were 79% more likely to have PMS than non-drinkers.

While other studies have found that even one glass of red wine can link in with GABA receptors and ease anxiety but other research has suggested that it could make symptoms worse.

Drinking alcohol affects the body's hormone levels. After drinking, multiple studies have measured increases in estrogen levels, and sometimes increases in testosterone and luteinizing hormone (LH). One particularly rigorous study examined how drinking affects hormone levels during different phases of the menstrual cycle. Multiple hormonal differences were measured, such as increases in androgen levels during the follicular phase, and increases in estrogen levels around ovulation, which persisted throughout the second half of the cycle. This effect has been shown to be stronger after binge drinking. However, the hormonal effects of moderate drinking did not lead to changes in menstrual cycle function.

My recommendation here is limit alcohol around your time of the month and the time of PMS, where possible. More research is needed on this area for a definitive answer. Drinking every so often won't have that much of an impact but if your PMS are difficult to manage alcohol may not be the best thing. Think everything in moderation.

Gut health

On the highest level, an imbalanced microbiome has been correlated with hormonal imbalances—and on the flip side, having too much estrogen in your body can cause gut-related issues like bloating and fluid retention.

So, if estrogen re-circulates through your body and

you develop excess levels of it, you'll probably experience symptoms pretty similar to PMS: heavier periods, bloating, mood swings, and more.

Fluctuating estrogen levels can impact the digestive tract, too, by leading to spasms in your intestines that can potentially cause diarrhoea. Or, you could have the opposite issue and experience constipation due to a dip in estrogen, which slows digestion.

The role of fibre cannot be downplayed when it comes to PMS and your cycle. If you are struggling to go to the bathroom your old estrogen (old cycle) has nowhere to go and painful periods may increase. But if you are ensuring that you are going to the bathroom regularly (ideally once a day or once every two days) this can help to ease PMS like symptoms.

Chia seeds, Flax seeds, fruit, whole grain carbs and vegetables will be very helpful.

If problems persist you may need the assistance of a probiotic but you will need to go to a doctor to get the correct strain of probiotic otherwise you don't know what you are taking and it may not have much impact.

Gut health is crucial for managing your PMS.

Caffeine

The American College of Obstetricians and Gynaecologists (ACOG) currently recommends that people who experience premenstrual syndrome

(PMS) avoid caffeine consumption, as evidence exists that women with PMS tend to consume more caffeine than those who do not. On the other hand, there are studies that suggest that there is no association.

Caffeine intake and PMS may be associated anecdotally and statistically, as fatigue and depression are common symptoms of PMS. In general, women in the luteal phase (the second half of the cycle, after ovulation) are found to have slower response time in cognitive tasks, and women with PMS performed worse on psychomotor tasks during their luteal phases as compared to during their follicular phases (the first half of their cycle, before and up to ovulation). These studies suggest that as women approach menstruation, they may experience fatigue and mental exhaustion, especially if they suffer from PMS.

People who experience fatigue may try to treat this symptom with increased caffeine consumption, leading to the reported association. Alternatively, women who consume high amounts of caffeine may also practice other behaviours, such as smoking, that are also associated with PMS, leading to a false association between caffeine intake and PMS.

It's difficult to say whether caffeine intake can actually cause PMS, because it's hard to prove that exposure to caffeine can lead to the outcome of PMS. Only one study has examined caffeine intake before diagnosis of PMS, and no association was found. Like with alcohol, think moderation when it comes to caffeine. Some women may have a higher caffeine threshold, meaning that they may be able to consume more than others.

If you struggle with sleep, caffeine has a life of 12 hours, meaning that if you drink caffeine at 11am it will still be in your body at 11pm. As a result, this could affect your sleep, mood, energy, appetite and overall increase PMS symptoms.

Keeping tabs on your symptoms can help you determine your typical premenstrual experience. If your symptoms are moderate to severe, it may be time to talk to your healthcare provider about exploring some potential causes for your symptoms and some more options for symptom relief.

Pain Management

Pain or discomfort is a very common symptom of PMS. Here are some common treatments for period pain that you may find useful:

Over the counter (OTC) medications

Over the counter medications such as Ibuprofen (Advil or Nurofen) help lower your body's production of prostaglandin which ultimately relieves period pain. It's important to be aware that relying on Ibuprofen is only a short-term solution and that once you find a more natural treatment you will probably find that you will not need these medications as often or at all.

Applying heat

Applying heat to your abdomen and lower back may relieve pain. A 2012 study focused on 147 women 18 to 30 years old who had regular menstrual cycles found that a heat patch at 104°F (40°C) was as effective as ibuprofen. You can use a hot water bottle, a heating pad or if you don't have either of those you can use a hot towel.

Massages

One 2010 study looked at 23 women with period pain caused by endometriosis. The researchers found that massages significantly reduced pain immediately and afterward.

Massage therapy for menstruation involves pressing specific points while the therapist's hands move around your abdomen, side, and back. The research would indicate that 20 minutes of massage therapy can help reduce menstrual pain.

If you add in some essential oils this has shown to have additional benefits.

Another study in 2012 divided 48 women experiencing menstrual pain into two groups: One group received a cream containing essential oils, while the other received a cream containing a synthetic fragrance.

The group who used essential oils experienced a significant reduction in amount and duration of pain.

Having an orgasm

While there are no clinical studies on the direct effect of orgasms on menstrual cramps, science suggests it may help.

A study carried out in 1985 by Dr. Beth Whipple was the first to find that vaginal self-stimulation doubled women's tolerance for pain.

Reducing certain foods

Reducing doesn't mean to take out or restrict (unless you have an intolerance or trying a FODMAP diet). Some foods can cause bloating and water retention. It is important to note that every women will be different when it comes to what foods may cause this, so it could be an idea to keep a log or a diary of the types of the foods that are causing the bloating and reduce these from there.

Some foods that can have this impact on people are:

- fatty foods
- alcohol
- carbonated beverages
- chewing gum
- caffeine
- salty foods

Adding herbs to your diet

Some experts believe that some herbal remedies contain anti-inflammatory and antispasmodic compounds that can reduce the muscle contractions and swelling associated with menstrual pain.

Some of these herbs include:

- *Chamomile tea* - A 2012 review of studies reports chamomile tea increases urinary levels of glycine, which helps relieve muscle spasms. Glycine also acts as a nerve relaxant. Sipping two cups of tea per day a week before your period may be of benefit.
- *Ginger* - One study of university students found that 250 mg of ginger powder four times a day for three days helped with pain relief. It also concluded ginger was as effective as ibuprofen. Start by grating a small piece of ginger into hot water for a warm cramp-relieving drink.
- *Dill* - A 2014 study concluded 1,000 mg dill was as effective for easing menstrual cramps as mefenamic acid, an OTC drug for menstrual pain. Try 1,000 mg of dill for five days, starting two days before your cycle.
- *Curcumin* (a natural chemical in turmeric) - may help with symptoms of premenstrual syndrome (PMS). One 2015 study looked at 70 women who took two capsules of curcumin for seven days before their period and three days after. Participants reported significant reduction in PMS.

Identify and treat histamine intolerance

Histamine intolerance is another cause of period

pain. It is caused by having too much of the inflammatory compound histamine. This could have an impact on headaches, anxiety, insomnia, brain fog and hives to name a few symptoms. It can also worsen period problems because it increases both inflammation and estrogen. PMS and period pain are two of the most common symptoms with histamine intolerance.

Migraines/Headaches

The effects can be different for every woman, so you may not experience the same changes as someone else.

If your headaches are hormonal in nature, you may find relief after menopause. This may mean that you have less headaches or less severe headaches. This is because your hormone levels stay low, with little fluctuation, after your period stops for good.

On the other hand, some women have more frequent or worse headaches during perimenopause. It's even possible for women who have never had problems with hormonal headaches to start having headaches during this time.

Women who experience migraines often report that their headaches are significantly worse during perimenopause.

Migraines are a subtype of headache. They're typically the most debilitating in nature. They're characterized by throbbing pain on one side of the head, as well as sensitivity to light or sound.

Estrogen withdrawal is a common trigger. This is why headaches can be worse around menstruation. The same hormone — or lack thereof — that gives some women relief from migraines after menopause can cause more headaches in the months leading up to it.

That's because hormone levels such as estrogen and progesterone decline during perimenopause. This decline isn't always consistent, so women who experience headaches related to their monthly menstrual cycle may have more headaches during perimenopause. It's also common to experience more severe headaches during this time.

If you are coming to the age of perimenopause and you suffer from migraines, please read the chapter on Menopause for more details.

<u>Diet changes</u>

What you eat can have a huge impact on your headaches. Keep in mind that what triggers your headaches won't be the same for someone else. Because of this, you may want to keep a food diary to determine what your headache triggers may be.

When you experience a headache, write down what you ate in the hours before. Over time this may help you find dietary patterns. If a pattern emerges, you should try limiting that item. From there, you can determine if cutting this out of your diet has an effect on your headaches.

Some of the most common dietary triggers I've seen with clients include:

- alcohol, especially red wine
- caffeine
- chocolate
- dairy products

Supplementation

Magnesium

According to a 2016 meta-analysis, magnesium is one of the best supplements for migraine prevention. A dose of 100mg -300mg will be the recommendation. Start on a lower dose and increase from there if needed. If you are on any medications please check with your doctor before taking it.

Vitamin b2 (riboflavin)

Vitamin b2 (riboflavin) has been clinically trialled for migraine prevention and found to reduce their frequency and was found to reduce their frequency by 50%. The dosage in the trials was 200mg twice per day.

Vitamin D and Coenzyme Q10 may also be beneficial. Taking ibuprofen short term could help manage the pain too. You should check with your doctor before adding these to your regimen to make sure you're not taking any unnecessary risks.

Exercise

Regular physical activity may also help to prevent headaches. Aim for 30 minutes of exercise three to four times each week. Spinning or swimming classes are two great choices. A nice walk outside is easy and accessible, too.

It's important to go slow in your activity goals. Let your body warm up gradually. Jumping into a high-intensity workout right away could actually trigger a headache.

Acupuncture

This is a form of alternative medicine that uses thin needles to stimulate your body's energy pathways. Acupuncture stems from traditional Chinese medicine and is used to treat various types of pain. Views on its effectiveness are mixed, but you may find that it helps you.

CBT

Cognitive behavioural therapy (CBT) is slightly different. CBT teaches you stress relief techniques, as well as how to better deal with stressors or pain. It's often recommended that you pair CBT with biofeedback or relaxation therapy for best results.

If you notice your headaches are becoming worse or interfering with your quality of life, you should speak with your doctor. They can rule out any other causes and, if necessary, adjust your treatment plan. Please note that you will need to always make sure you're buying herbs and supplements from a reputable source as they aren't regulated. While most of these herbal remedies are great some may have some side effects, check with your doctor before trying them as some can have unintended side effects with certain medications.

Managing your change in Mood

This section of the book is so important and discusses how to manage the change in moods at certain times of the month.

In the amazing book by Red School entitled "Wild Power" they talk about the various stages of the cycle as if comparing it to the seasons of the year. They call this concept the Map of your Inner seasons or the Four Seasons of the Menstrual Cycle.

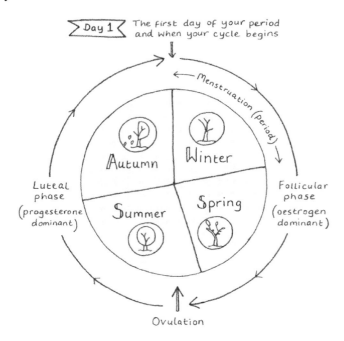

Please note: This idea does not have any evidence to it but it is an amazing concept that

allows clients to understand and link in with how they are feeling around certain times of the month.

Like the seasons of the year, through your menstrual month you move through an inner winter, spring, summer and autumn and back to winter again. Each phase ushers in a set of very specific resources and psychological challenges. To give you a rough idea of these phases, in a classic 28-day cycle:

- The inner winter is approximately day 27 to day 5
- The inner spring is approximately day 6 to day 11
- The inner summer is approximately day 12 to day 19
- The inner autumn approximately day 20 to day 26

However, do not get too hung up on exact days. The important thing is to sense and follow your own cycle experience, and discover the season changing moments for yourself. As you bring consciousness to and care for each season in turn, you restore the order of the cycle, your inner ecology, and with that create a feeling of greater ease and pleasure, coherence and effectiveness in using your power.

So, let's look into the seasons in a little bit more detail:

Season: Winter
Menstrual Phase

Winter is a time of inward reflection, a time of metaphorical death.

The bleeding phase of your cycle is the time where your energy and hormones are at an all-time low. Most women when left to their own devices will take more rest on the first few days of their moon time.

Hibernation and rest are two qualities that accurately characterize what this phase is about for a woman. As a woman moves into her inner winter, she might find it irritating when family members, partners or friends are asking her to "do things" for them during this phase. Winter is not a time to give to others, but to yourselves. Learning to be self-loving during this time is the healthiest behaviour you can adopt for ourselves and our families. Taking baths, having movie nights at home with your partner, spending the days alone creating or writing/reading in bed, sleeping, and being in nature.

Season: Spring
Follicular Phase

Think rebirth, renew, fresh-start, cleansed, energized and happy. As a woman moves into her inner Spring phase, she's ready to get back into the world slowly and take on new projects, start planning and organizing your month.

During this phase, the hormone estradiol (an

estrogen) is rising and energy levels start making a comeback. This is an optimal time to dedicate focused time to projects, reading and researching, learning, and performing physical tasks. You might find this is the best time to move, or to take on a challenge.

Season: Summer
<u>Ovulation Phase</u>

This is the third week of the menstrual cycle, where ovulation occurs.

A woman with a 29.5-day cycle may ovulate on the 14th day, though some will ovulate a bit earlier or later.

You may feel more social, and this is a great time to focus on community building, nurturing relationships, hosting, cooking or being of service to others. Summer week is the most enjoyable time for taking care of children, offering friends support and having lots of delicious sex with your partner, with caution of course, because while pleasure is heightened at this time, so is your fertility. Oh, and by the way, some research suggests that ovulation is the best time to ask for what you want – whether that be from your partner, or asking for a raise at work.

Season: Autumn
Luteal Phase

Autumn is the fourth week of your cycle, and this is where things start winding down.

A woman might notice herself feeling more inward at this time. She may become agitated by excessive demands placed upon her, craving more spaciousness and time alone. It is important to schedule your life and routine around your cycle and purposefully schedule days off leading up to your cycle, dedicating time to self-care. I encourage the women I coach and mentor to do the same. If you disown your own needs, PMS may intensify and wreak havoc in your lives.

Choosing consciously to acknowledge this inward phase is a courageous act of self-love.

When to see your doctor

It is important to note that these may appear at various stages of the cycle and being in-tune with your body could help you to understand your body for you and it could help you to bring you closer to your partner so that they can understand how you feel at various times. Natural cycles is the best way to keep a log of what week you are on but there are apps like Kindara and Clue that are also very useful.

This amazing concept is not evidence based but is based on the psychological aspect of PMS with the imagery of the four seasons of the year. This week may be different for every woman so it is important that you keep a log of when you notice when you can take on the world and notice when you may need to take a self-care day.

Nutrition and PMS

Many can struggle with many of the symptoms that have been mentioned throughout the chapter. But all is not lost and there are things you can implement for you and your clients nutritionally and these include looking at the types of foods you are consuming and some foods that may not be of benefit to you. The following list is not a complete list and some women may have intolerances or may benefit from looking into a FODMAP diet if you struggle with IBS.

Foods to include:

Water

Drinking a lot of water is always important, and this is especially true during your period. Staying hydrated can reduce your chances of getting dehydration headaches, a common symptom of menstruation.

Drinking plenty of water can also stop you from retaining water and bloating. Think of water as your new best friend around this time. It will really help to reduce any bloating and will also help to help with your digestion.

Fruit

Water-rich fruits, such as watermelon and cucumber, are great for staying hydrated. Sweet fruits can help you curb your cravings. An amazing recipe that I recommend every woman tries around this time of the month is Greek Yoghurt, x2 squares dark chocolate, Chia Seeds, Flax Seeds, Blueberries and throw it into a bowl and all I can say is watch your life change.

Leafy green vegetables

It's common to experience a dip in your iron levels during your period, particularly if your menstrual flow is heavy. This can lead to fatigue, bodily pain, and dizziness.

Leafy green vegetables such as kale and spinach can boost your iron levels. Spinach is also rich in magnesium. If you are deficient in iron, it is essential that you get your bloods checked and your doctor will provide you with adequate supplementation. I highly encourage getting your blood and hormones screened on a regular basis.

Ginger

A warm mug of ginger tea can improve certain symptoms of menstruation. Ginger has anti-inflammatory effects, which can soothe achy muscles.

Ginger may also reduce nausea. There are a few studies that confirm this, but a 2018 study found that ginger effectively reduced nausea and vomiting during the first trimester of pregnancy. Since it's safe and relatively cheap, it's worth trying.

Don't consume too much ginger, though: Consuming more than 4 grams in one day could cause heartburn and stomach aches.

Protein

Think protein. No, you will not turn into Arnie or the Rock by consuming protein. Eating protein is essential for your overall health, and it can help you stay full and satiated during your period, curbing cravings. It will also help you to improve overall bone health and help you to build muscle.

Fish

Rich in iron, protein, and omega-3 fatty acids, fish is a nutritious addition to your diet. Consuming iron will counteract the dip in iron levels that you might experience while menstruating.

Omega-3s can reduce the intensity of period pain, according to a 2012 study. Subjects who took omega-3 supplements found that their menstrual pain decreased so much that they could reduce the amount of ibuprofen they took.

A 2014 study showed that omega-3s can also reduce depression. For those who experience mood swings and depression around menstruation, omega-3s may be helpful.

Turmeric

Turmeric is known as an anti-inflammatory spice, and curcumin is its main active ingredient. A 2015 study looked at the effects of curcumin on PMS symptoms and found that people who took curcumin had less severe symptoms.

Dark chocolate (yes you read right)

A tasty and beneficial snack, dark chocolate is rich in iron and magnesium. A 100-gram bar of 70 to 85 percent dark chocolate contains 67 percent of the recommended daily intake (RDI) for iron and 58 percent of the RDI for magnesium.

A 2010 study found that magnesium reduced the severity of PMS symptoms. According to a 2015 study, people with magnesium deficiencies were more likely to have severe PMS symptoms.

I encourage all of my clients to have chocolate every day. If you restrict yourself, you won't last very long. Think of chocolate as a soul food, it's good for the soul.

Nuts

Most nuts are rich in omega-3 fatty acids. They also contain magnesium and various vitamins. If you don't want to eat nuts on their own, try nut butters or nut-based milks or add these ingredients to smoothies. Please be mindful that nuts are higher in calories than other foods and the calories in them can add up quite easily.

Flaxseed oil

A small study found that consuming flaxseed oil soothed constipation, a common symptom of menstruation. However, more research is needed to show how flaxseed oil can improve digestive health.

Quinoa

Quinoa is rich in nutrients such as iron, protein, and magnesium. It's also gluten-free, so it's a great food for those with celiac disease. Plus, it has a low glycemic index, which means you're likely to feel full and have energy for a long time after eating it.

Lentils and beans

Lentils and beans are rich in protein, so they're good meat replacements for vegans and vegetarians. They're also rich in iron, which makes them great additions to your diet if your iron levels are low.

Yogurt

Many people get yeast infections during or after their period. If you tend to get yeast infections, probiotic-rich foods like yogurt can nourish the "good" bacteria in your vagina and may help you fight the infections.

Yogurt is also rich in magnesium and other essential nutrients, like calcium.

Tofu

A popular source of protein for vegetarians and vegans, tofu is made from soybeans. It's rich in iron, magnesium, and calcium.

Peppermint tea

A 2016 study suggests that peppermint tea can soothe the symptoms of PMS. Specifically, it can relieve menstrual cramps, nausea, and diarrhoea.

Kombucha

Yogurt isn't the only probiotic-rich food with yeast-fighting benefits. If you're avoiding dairy, kombucha tea is a great fermented food that's more widely available than ever before.

Whole Grain Carbs

Before I write anything, it is important to note that there is nothing wrong with white carbohydrates; they just may not be the most beneficial during PMS. That's not to say don't eat everything in moderation. The reason for suggesting whole grain carbs over white carbs would be for digestion but also to regulate blood sugars.

White carbs can spike up blood sugars and drop them down quite quickly but with whole grain carbs, blood sugars remain steadier and you won't be as hungry as quickly.

So, think wholegrain where possible.

When you are thinking about foods, think inclusive. There is no need to remove any foods from your life, unless there is an allergy or you suffer from IBS. The foods listed below are foods to watch out for and eat in moderation:

Salt

Consuming lots of salt leads to water retention, which can result in bloating. To reduce bloating, don't add salt to your foods and avoid highly processed foods that contain a lot of sodium.

Highly processed foods

It's OK to have processed foods in moderation, but eating too much of it can cause a spike in energy followed by a crash. This can worsen your mood. If you tend to feel moody, depressed, or anxious during your period, watching your processed foods intake can help regulate your mood.

I normally suggest to clients to have a date or family night once a week where they are present and have a takeaway if they so wish.

Coffee

Caffeine can cause water retention and bloating. It can also exacerbate headaches. But caffeine withdrawal can cause headaches, too, so don't cut out coffee completely if you're used to having a few cups a day.

Coffee might also cause digestive issues. If you tend to get diarrhoea during your period, reducing your coffee intake could stop this from happening (see the section on caffeine for more information).

Alcohol

Alcohol can have a number of negative effects on your body, which can exacerbate the symptoms of your period.

For example, alcohol can dehydrate you, which can worsen headaches and cause bloating. It can also lead to digestive issues, such as diarrhoea and nausea.

Plus, a hangover can bring on some of the same symptoms that occur during your period, including:

- headaches
- nausea
- vomiting
- diarrhoea
- Fatigue

Spicy foods

Many people find that spicy foods upset their stomachs, giving them diarrhoea, stomach pain, and even nausea. If your stomach struggles to tolerate spicy foods or if you're not used to eating them, it might be best to avoid them during your period. I would watch out for spicy foods if you are finding that you are suffering from hot flashes.

Foods you don't tolerate well

This might seem obvious, but it's worth emphasizing: If you have food sensitivities, avoid those foods, especially during your period.

Eating these foods can cause nausea, constipation, or diarrhoea, which will only add to your discomfort when you're having a painful period. Keep a diary of these foods and over time you will be able to spot a trend of what food causes what symptom.

Managing your Cravings

It's common to have cravings during or after your period. Progesterone, a hormone that is at its peak just before your period, is associated with a bigger appetite, according to a 2011 study. As such, you might feel hungrier at that time.

Plus, if your mood is low, you might feel the need for comfort food. Eat the foods you enjoy, but remember that moderation is key.

Stop apologizing for wanting some chocolate or carbs just before your period.

Period cravings and hunger are real and there are reasons — legitimate, scientifically proven reasons — why you want to eat all the things before your period.

Why does it happen?

Hormones play a major role in an individual's menstrual cycle, but aren't the only reason for bad premenstrual moods. Overall mental and physical health have a greater impact on mood than the menstrual cycle phase.

Your body releases serotonin when you eat starchy foods and sweets. Serotonin is a chemical that boosts feelings of happiness. A boost in good feelings is always nice, but even more so when you have PMS-like symptoms. This explains why when you are in a lower mood that your brain kicks in and searches for the types of foods mentioned above.

But there could be something else at play, and that is your emotions. Cravings are totally normal and can arise for a number of different reasons due to complex interactions between our bodies, brains and the environment we live in.

Experiencing cravings doesn't make you a bad person. It actually makes you human.

How early can the cravings start?

Period-related cravings usually start around 7 to 10 days before your period starts. This is also when other PMS symptoms tend to start, like changes to your bowel habits, headaches, acne, and bloating.

The urge to stuff one's face usually disappears once your period starts.

Is it OK to indulge?

YES! It's not just OK, but it's important to listen to your body before your period.

Certain cravings may be happening for a reason, and your body may need more calories. The research states giving your body an extra 200-300 extra calories for the days around this time. If you are counting calories this is a rough guide. If you are not counting calories I would aim to include a little more at meals or include some more dark chocolate.

There is magnesium in dark chocolate which can help manage PMS. Supplementing with Magnesium is highly recommended around this time and continuously throughout your month.

This isn't to say that you should be overindulging on the daily, of course. But, if your body's begging you for something different ahead of your period, don't beat yourself up for eating more than you might normally.

Paying attention to your body and its needs is key.

Your body could be trying to tell you something also. Around this time is when the negative voice can speak up and more self-esteem issues, body image issues or lower mood may happen.

Try to keep a continuous log of how you feel around this time. You may notice a trend of the same things cropping up over and over. If you are finding that when this negative voice speaks up make a log of how you feel before the food and write down how you feel.

An example of a worksheet that I use with clients is below:

Food'n'Mood

Date: _____ Mon Tue Wed Thurs Fri Sat Sun   Weight: _____

Check # 8 ounce glasses of water ☐ ☐ ☐ ☐ ☐ ☐ ☐

Time	Place	Food/Beverage	How Much	Mood Before	Mood After

What's your Mood: peaceful, angry, sad, frustrated, obsessed, depressed, overwhelmed, anxious, lonely, jealous, worried, hopeful, in love, happy, thrilled, etc.

My Day in Review: (Times/situations/moods likely to cause cravings, types of food most likely to crave, etc.)
_____
_____

Behaviors that require my attention: _____
_____

Notes: _____
_____

How to use the Journal?

The secret behind this is to implement a pause (20-30 mins is normally advised). For example, if you notice a trend that when you are in a lower mood or stressed that you are finding yourself eating more processed food or picking more than usual then the pausing and journal can really help you to understand how you cope with your emotions.

It's important to note that we all emotionally eat. Emotional eating is also a positive thing, look at Christmas and birthdays.

The only time that I would look into negative emotions and eating is if food is the coping mechanism all the time for this emotion, e.g., stress or loneliness. This exercise can be really helpful but can take time to implement so please be patient and realise it won't happen every time. If it reduces the eating by even 1% it's a huge step.

The foods I eat just make me feel worse!

Yeah, that tends to happen when we eat foods high in refined sugar, salt, and carbs.

Swapping out what you're craving for healthier alternatives or limiting portions of those crave-able items can help give your body what it's screaming for without making you feel worse.

If it's carbs you crave

Reaching for simple carbs when you're feeling tired

can make you feel better because of the increase in serotonin, but the effect is short lived. Have too many and you could end up feeling even more sluggish.

Instead of simple carbs, like chips, bread, or pasta, choose complex carbs (whole grain) that increase serotonin but make you feel fuller for longer. These include things like beans and lentils, brown rice, and oats.

It's important to note that carbs are not bad for you! In fact, they are quite the opposite. They are the key that start your engine, a.k.a ovulation. Without the necessary carbs you don't ovulate.

<u>If you've just got to satisfy a sweet tooth</u>

Tempting as it may be to eat an entire bag of Oreos when your sweet tooth is begging for satisfaction, too much sugar usually leads to a pretty unpleasant crash.

Go ahead and have a cookie or two if you feel inclined. However, there are other ways to satisfy a craving.

Some alternative ideas:

- smoothies
- fruit and yogurt
- apple slices drizzled with honey
- energy bites
- trail mix

It's important to note that sugar craving is not a thing. It could be a sign of something else. Our bodies can't say I crave a certain food. How often has your body said "I crave a pavlova". There could be something else emotionally going on and using a tool like the journal could really help you to discover what's going on.

When it comes to food cravings, you probably fall into one of two categories. You might crave sweet things like cookies or chocolate. Or you might crave a big bag of potato chips or salty pretzels. Maybe you crave both? But a lot can be said about the types of food you crave.

So, are you a sweet or savoury woman?

The reasons we crave more processed foods are partly physiological, partly psychological and partly because of the environment in which we live.

The human body functions a bit like a car – you put fuel in the tank, and then you drive. If the body doesn't get the fuel it needs, then strong physical cravings can manifest.

What kind of fuel does your body need? A balanced intake throughout the day of high-fibre carbohydrates, lean protein and heart-healthy fats.

These three factors that can contribute to cravings:

You're starving/restricting yourself

Think you're being "good" by having coffee for

breakfast and a garden salad for lunch?

Truly, you're setting yourself up for failure in the afternoon and evening. If you go too long without eating, your body will crave the fastest fuel it can think of — refined grains and simple sugars. These are also known as empty carbs such as chips, as well as candy and cookies.

Another popular trap you may be guilty of is meal-skipping or waiting too long between meals to eat. This leads to significant hunger, which makes you crave anything sweet or salty you can get your hands on.

Having an all-or-nothing mentality — forbidding all foods with sugar or salt — can backfire too.

Why do you crave more processed food?

For one thing, they taste good. Many food companies conduct research to determine which food components will tempt consumers' taste buds the most.

Our brains are wired to enjoy things which make us happy. Sugar, in particular, releases brain chemicals, like serotonin, that make us feel good. This leaves us wanting to experience that good feeling over and over again, day after day.

Many people say they're 'sugar addicts,' consuming real sugar and artificial sweeteners in various forms. But it's not the sugar itself you are addicted to, it's the chemical trigger in the brain or the emotional trigger that it relieves.

You're not listening to your body

Jonesing for a sweet or salt? Before you indulge, check your fatigue level. Research shows that when you're tired, you're more likely to turn to whatever you crave to get more energy or to wake up.

Perhaps you find yourself over indulging on salty snacks. The next time it happens, pay attention to your stress levels. Stress may impair your adrenal glands' ability to regulate sodium, which may lead to salt cravings. (This would be the ideal time to use the Food and Mood journal mentioned previously)

Take thirst into account, too. Some research suggests that mistaking dehydration for hunger may trigger cravings as well.

Finally, if you have diabetes, you probably know you get hungrier than other people. But excessive hunger can mean your blood sugar is too high or too low.

Chocolate is life!

Chocolate is one of the most common foods craved by people before their periods. Lucky for you, there are benefits to chocolate.

Stick to dark chocolate if you want to reap the real health benefits of this craving. Dark chocolate's high in antioxidants and minerals and just a square or two of high-quality dark chocolate can often do the trick.

You are probably eating the chocolate anyway. The only difference with what I'm suggesting is giving yourself unconditional permission to do it. If the same emotion is constantly coming up then you need to look at the emotion that is present.

Ask yourself this very important question:

"What is the third or fourth bar/square doing that the first one didn't?"

Overeating and emotional eating will happen, you are human. If it's getting to the point of where you have no control and can't stop (definition of a binge) then please talk to your doctor, dietician or a mental health professional. Some accounts who I highly encourage to follow on social media are Jamie Wright **@jamiesdietguide**, Emilia Thompson **@emiliathompsonphd**, **@bodywhys** and **@break.binge.eating**. These accounts provide amazing content on emotional eating and eating disorders.

Instead of trying to stuff all the feelings down with a fistful of gummy bears, try activities that have been proven to increase your body's happy hormones: endorphins, serotonin, oxytocin, and dopamine.

By all means, keep eating those gummy bears, just make sure you're doing something else for your emotional health.

If you want to improve your mood and increase your energy, you can:

- take a walk
- go for a run
- have sex — partnered or solo
- watch a funny movie
- talk to a friend
- cuddle your pet

<u>When to see a doctor</u>

Wanting to eat more than usual before your period and having cravings is pretty common and not usually anything to worry about.

That said, there are some circumstances that could indicate an underlying issue.

See your doctor if your hunger or cravings:

- persist throughout the month
- are a way to cope with persistent or severe feelings of depression, anxiety, or stress
- lead to significant weight gain
- cause you anxiety or distress
- impact your treatment or recovery from an eating disorder
- interfere with your ability to perform at school or work

Rest assured you're not the only one grabbing every snack in your press before your period.

Instead of beating yourself up over your cravings, listen to your body and give it what it needs.

If that means that once a month it needs pizza and ice cream, then so be it.

Think wholegrain, more regular meals, chocolate, fruit, protein and increase calories by 200-300 if you feel you need it or if you need more go for it.

Common Myths about PMS

Myth #1: All women and people with cycles have PMS

This myth comes from the popular misconception that any symptoms that occur before the period are directly related to PMS. In truth, just because a person experiences some premenstrual symptoms does not mean they have PMS.

While some people might experience premenstrual symptoms of low to moderate intensity, if they don't have a significant negative effect on a person's life, this is not considered PMS (from a medical perspective).

Reported rates of PMS vary so widely that it's nearly impossible to say how many people experience it. This is probably because PMS is sometimes used as a catch-all term for experiencing any premenstrual symptoms, and not only the diagnosis of PMS.

Many people who use the phrase "PMS" to define

their premenstrual experiences are referring to their cluster of individual symptoms, rather than a medical diagnosis. For example, a headache that happens a few days before a person's period might not have a significant negative impact on their day-to-day functioning, even though it's uncomfortable. In this case, the headache is a mild premenstrual symptom. A recurrent experience of depression, insomnia, and extreme fatigue, on the other hand, might significantly impact someone's well-being and therefore meet the criteria for PMS or even premenstrual dysphoric disease (PMDD).

Myth #2: The premenstrual phase is all about bad moods

Science supports that the premenstrual experience is not inherently negative for everyone, despite what culture, society and media suggest. Culturally and socially it's more common to talk about negative premenstrual experiences, but this limits the true experience of the premenstrual phase, because it includes positive factors as well.

Current research has primarily connected negative moods to biological mechanisms, like hormone fluctuations. Most PMS research has deduced a linear relationship between biology and behaviour, and failed to reflect the real experience of PMS within a socio-cultural context.

Researchers have pointed out that many of the studies of PMS suffer from major methodological errors. It was reported that in many studies, research participants were asked about their mood but were given a list to choose from that only included negative options. If researchers only study negative moods, it doesn't accurately reflect the experience of PMS.

Without clear scientific evidence, why is the idea of negative premenstrual mood so pervasive?

It boils down to cultural perceptions of menstruation. People who are socialized to expect a negative premenstrual experience are primed to report more problems, contributing to negative attitudes towards the cycle.

PMS is not a one-size-fits all experience, rather, each person's experience is filtered through social and cultural beliefs that influence how they process symptoms.

Track your symptoms and your cycle and you will spot a pattern over time. Try tracking your cycle for 3 months as a starting point.

Myth #3: Bad moods in your premenstrual phase can be blamed exclusively on hormone fluctuations.

Hormones play a major role in an individual's menstrual cycle, but aren't the only reason for negative premenstrual moods. Overall mental and physical health has a greater impact on mood than the menstrual cycle phase.

Participants of a recent study tracked daily mood and health data over six months to test a commonly stated fact amongst researchers that the premenstrual phase is the source of depressed, irritable moods and mood swings. The study tracked both positive and negative moods, collected data from every cycle phase (not just the premenstrual phase) and followed several consecutive menstrual cycles.

The conclusion was surprising; data did not support the idea of a negative mood prevailing in the premenstrual phase. Social support, physical health, and perceived stress were more significant as predictors of daily mood than menstrual cycle phase.

Still, it could be true that hormones may be the cause of premenstrual syndrome for some people. Lower levels of estrogen in the premenstrual phase may cause decreased levels of serotonin and dampened mood. More research is needed on this.

Conclusion

Every woman is so different with symptoms and the management of them. Try to track your cycle and log what symptoms are coming up regularly and note that it could be a simple lifestyle change like managing stress. If you have a more severe form called PMDD it is important you know that the proper support is out there through CBT or counselling or medication.

Please check with your doctor before taking certain supplements as they may interact with certain medications. Please do not take all of them together either.

PMS can be managed. It's about knowing what's causing it and then you can live the life you always wanted.

Chapter 3 – The Pill

Women's health and female empowerment is at an all-time high and it's amazing to see, and long may it continue. So many more women are taking control of their bodies and understanding how their bodies work for them. One of the biggest topics right now is whether women should take the pill or should stop it completely.

Women have faced a long history of discrimination when it comes to birth control. Up until the mid-20th century, women were largely expected to stay at home and produce children whilst their husbands were out at work. They had little control over when they became pregnant or even over their own bodies.

Something needed to change.

After being created in the late 1940s in Mexico City by Dr Carl Djerassi, it took a while for the other governments like those in the UK and Ireland to take notice.

The pill was first introduced in the UK in the early 1960's after clinical trials in London, Birmingham and Slough. Around this time, the UK health minister Enoch Powell announced that married women who wished to use oral contraceptives would be able access it through the NHS.

At first, contraception advice was only given to older

married women who no longer wanted children, or to those whose health would be at serious risk during pregnancy. In 1967 the NHS Family Planning Act 1967 was passed, which recognised that unwanted children in low-income households caused a serious financial strain for those families. As a result, the oral contraceptive pill became more widely available on the NHS, and the FPA (Family Planning Association) were able to approve the use of it in their clinics.

In Ireland a highly controversial vote on February 20, 1985, the Irish government defied the powerful Catholic Church and approved the sale of contraceptives. Up until 1979, Irish law prohibited the importation and sale of contraceptives. As you can see it has not been very long since these bans were lifted and only now is more information being put out there for women.

These have both been radical movements for women and it can't just stop there!

Birth control

The type of birth control you use is a personal decision, and there are many options to choose from. If you're a sexually active female, you may consider birth control pills or get your partner to consider using condoms.

Birth control pills, also called oral contraceptives, are medications you take by mouth to prevent pregnancy. They're an effective method of birth control. Knowing how the various types of birth control affect your body cannot be downplayed.

It is important to communicate with your partner and if you feel comfortable to do so with family on the decision. You ultimately have final say as it's your body, don't forget that!

Please note: You will not ovulate if you are on the Pill which may prevent pregnancy but can come with other caveats including bone density in later life.

It is important to know what you are putting into your body and be aware of what each pill/contraception does and the impact it has on your body. They are not real hormones so will not be better than your own hormones. They are not as good as the real thing for your body.

What are the different types of birth control?

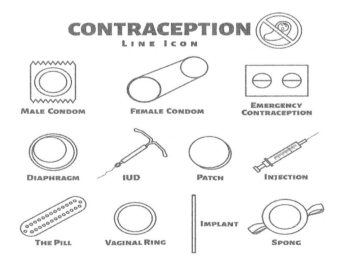

Combination pills

Combination pills contain synthetic (man-made) forms of the hormones estrogen (estradiol) and progestin. It's important to note that progestin isn't the same as your hormones Progesterone. I compare this to putting unleaded petrol into a diesel car.

Progesterone is the naturally occurring hormone in the body, which originates from the ovaries and has various duties in the reproduction and menstruation cycles. Progestin is a synthetic, lab created hormone that is meant to mimic progesterone and act as it does in the body. The main difference between the two is that progesterone is naturally occurring and, while progestin is similar but not identical.

Most pills in each cycle are active, which means they contain hormones. The remaining pills are inactive, which means they don't contain hormones. There are several types of combination pills:

Monophasic pills:

These are used in one-month cycles and each active pill gives you the same dose of hormone. During the last week of the cycle, you take inactive pills and have your period.

Multiphasic pills:

These are used in one-month cycles and provide

different levels of hormones during the cycle. During the last week of the cycle, you take inactive pills and have your period.

Extended-cycle pills:

These are typically used in 13-week cycles. You take active pills for 12 weeks, and during the last week of the cycle, you take inactive pills and have your period. As a result, you have your period only three to four times per year.

Examples of brand-name combination pills include the likes of Azurette, Beyaz, Levora, Yasmin, Brenda and Yaz.

Progestin-only pills or Mini Pill

Progestin-only pills contain progestin without estrogen. This type of pill is also called the mini pill. Progestin-only pills may be a good choice for women who can't take estrogen for health or other reasons. With these progestin-only pills, all pills in the cycle are active. There are no inactive pills, so you may or may not have a period while taking progestin-only pills.

Examples of progestin-only pills include Camila, Errin, Heather, Jencycla, Nor-QD and Ortho Micronor.

NuvaRing (vaginal ring)

The vaginal ring (NuvaRing) is a small soft, plastic ring that you place inside your vagina.

It releases a continuous dose of the hormones estrogen and progestogen into the bloodstream to prevent pregnancy. If used correctly, the vaginal ring is more than 99% effective.

The ring steadily releases the hormones estrogen and progestogen into your bloodstream, which prevents the release of an egg each month.

It also thickens the cervical mucus, which makes it more difficult for sperm to move through the cervix, and thins the lining of the womb so a fertilised egg is less likely to implant itself.

You can start using the vaginal ring at any time during your menstrual cycle if you're not pregnant.

The standard way to use the ring is you leave it in for 21 days, then remove it and have a 7-day ring-free break. You're protected against pregnancy during the ring-free break. After the 7-day break you then put a new ring in for another 21 days.

You can also choose to have a shorter ring-free break or not to have a break at all. You'll be protected against pregnancy straight away if you insert it in the first 5 days of your period (the first 5 days of your menstrual cycle). Talk to a GP or nurse about whether you need additional contraception if you have a very short cycle or an irregular cycle.

Some evidence has shown that the NuvaRing comes with a higher risk of blood clots because the ethinylestradiol goes directly into the blood without first passing through your liver. This should be discussed in detail with your doctor when discussing your options.

Contraceptive patch

The contraceptive patch is a small sticky patch that releases similar hormones to that of the combined pill. In the UK and Ireland, the patch's brand name is Evra.
When used correctly, the patch is more than 99% effective at preventing pregnancy.
Each patch lasts for 1 week. You change the patch every week for 3 weeks, then have a week off without a patch. If you have heavy or painful periods, the patch can help.

The patch releases a daily dose of hormones through the skin into the bloodstream to prevent pregnancy. It contains the same hormones as the combined pill – estradiol and progestin – and works in the same way by preventing the release of an egg each month (ovulation).

It is important to note that the patch can raise your blood pressure, and some women get temporary side effects, such as headaches. Some women develop a blood clot and it may not be suitable for women who smoke, are 35 or over, or who weigh over 90kg (14 stone).

It is important to note that the patch does not protect against sexually transmitted infections (STIs), so you may need to use condoms as well.

A very small number of people using the patch may develop a blood clot in a vein or an artery. Don't use the patch if you've had a blood clot before.

Contraceptive implant

The contraceptive implant (Nexplanon) is a small flexible plastic rod that's placed under the skin in your upper arm by a doctor or nurse.

It releases the hormone progestin into your bloodstream to prevent pregnancy and lasts for 3 years. They contain either the progestin levonorgestrel or etonogestrel. It also thickens the cervical mucus, which makes it more difficult for sperm to move through the cervix, and thins the lining of the womb so a fertilised egg is less likely to implant itself.

It can be useful for women who can't use contraception that contains estrogen. The implant can be taken out if you have side effects. It's very useful for women who find it difficult to remember to take a pill at the same time every day. A common side effect is that your periods stop (amenorrhoea). It's not harmful, but you may want to consider this before deciding to have an implant.

One of the common things that is seen is your periods may become irregular, lighter, heavier or longer, so it's important to talk to your GP if this is happening. Please check out the chapter on these symptoms later on in the book.

Injection (Progestin-Only)

The contraceptive injection (Depo-Provera, Sayana Press or Noristerat) releases the hormone progestogen into your bloodstream to prevent pregnancy. Depo-Provera is most commonly given and lasts for 13 weeks. Occasionally, Noristerat may be given, which lasts for 8 weeks.

The contraceptive injection steadily releases the hormone progestogen into your bloodstream, which prevents the release of an egg each month (ovulation).

It also thickens the cervical mucus, which makes it difficult for sperm to move through the cervix, and thins the lining of the womb so a fertilised egg is less likely to implant itself.

You usually have the Depo-Provera and Noristerat injections in your bottom, but you can have them in your upper arm.

You can have the Sayana Press injection in your tummy (abdomen) or thigh and would normally learn to do this yourself.

There's a small risk of infection at the site of the injection. In very rare cases, some people may have an allergic reaction to the injection.

Using Depo-Provera affects your natural estrogen levels, which can cause thinning of the bones, but it does not increase your risk of breaking a bone.

This is not a problem for most women because the bone replaces itself when you stop the injection, and it does not appear to cause any long-term problems. Another thing to note is that some people may put on weight when they use Depo-Provera or Sayana Press contraceptive injections. This will not be fat gain. Please check later on in the chapter for more information on the link between weight gain and the pill.

Some research shows that it can be associated with an increase in breast cancer risk.

Sometimes the doctor may recommend that you stop after 2 years so there's no long-term effect on your bones. It's very useful for women who find it difficult to remember to take a pill at the same time every day.

Hormonal IUD (Mirena and Skyla)

Mirena and Skyla are hormonal intrauterine devices (IUD) that can provide long-term birth control (contraception).

The device is a T-shaped plastic frame that's inserted into the uterus, where it releases a type of the hormone progestin. To prevent pregnancy, they thicken mucus in the cervix to stop sperm from reaching or fertilizing an egg and thin the lining of the uterus and partially suppresses ovulation but not as often as other progestin only methods. The hormonal IUD suppresses ovulation in 85% of cycles in the first year, but then only 15% of cycles after that.

There has been some research that the hormonal IUD has been linked to depression and may reduce your ability to cope with stress, more research is needed on this for a definitive link.

Because of these non-contraceptive benefits, Mirena is often prescribed for women with:

- Heavy menstrual bleeding
- Cramping or pain with periods
- Endometriosis
- Abnormal growth of the lining of the uterus (endometrial hyperplasia)
- Abnormal growth of uterine-lining tissue into the muscular wall of the uterus (adenomyosis)
- Anaemia
- Fibroids

Mirena isn't appropriate for everyone.

Your health care provider may discourage use of Mirena if you have:

- Breast cancer (check if cancer is in the family), or have had it
- Uterine or cervical cancer
- Liver disease
- Uterine abnormalities, such as fibroids, that interfere with the placement or retention of Mirena
- A pelvic infection or current pelvic inflammatory disease
- Unexplained vaginal bleeding

Tell your health care provider if you:

- Take any medications, including non-prescription and herbal products
- Have diabetes or high blood pressure
- Have a heart condition or have had a heart attack
- Have migraines
- Have blood-clotting problems or have had a stroke
- Recently gave birth or are breast-feeding

With most hormonal birth control, you bleed but don't get a cycle. With the Mirena IUD, you cycle but you don't bleed. As the Mirena does not completely suppress ovulation it may be the least harmful of all birth control.

Copper IUD

An IUD is a small T-shaped plastic and copper device that's put into your womb (uterus) by a doctor or nurse.

It releases copper to stop you getting pregnant, and protects against pregnancy for between 5 and 10 years. It's sometimes called a "coil" or "copper coil". An IUD can be fitted at any time during your menstrual cycle, as long as you're not pregnant. You'll be protected against pregnancy straight away.

The IUD is similar to the intrauterine system (IUS), but instead of releasing the hormone progestogen like the IUS, the IUD release copper into the womb.

The copper alters the cervical mucus, which makes it more difficult for sperm to reach an egg and survive. It can also stop a fertilised egg from being able to implant itself.

If you're 40 or over when you have an IUD fitted, it can be left in until you reach the menopause or you no longer need contraception.

Your IUD can be removed at any time by a trained doctor or nurse.

If you're not having another IUD put in and do not want to get pregnant, use additional contraception, such as condoms, for 7 days before you have it removed.

It's possible to get pregnant as soon as the IUD has been taken out.

Two of the major advantages of using the non-hormonal IUD is there are no hormonal side effects, such as acne, headaches or breast tenderness and there's no evidence that an IUD will affect your weight or increase the risk of cervical cancer, womb (uterus) cancer or ovarian cancer.
There are a couple of warnings with this method that your periods can be heavier, longer or more painful in the first 3 to 6 months after an IUD is put in. You might get spotting or bleeding between periods. The other one is that there's a small chance that the IUD can be rejected (expelled) by the womb or it can move (displacement).

If you're suffering from bloating it is a normal side

effect. But if it is occurring 6 months after insertion it could do no harm in talking to your doctor to see if everything is ok and it hasn't been displaced.

If this happens, it's usually soon after it's been fitted. You'll be taught how to check that your IUD is in place.

Condom

Condoms are the **only** type of contraception that can both prevent pregnancy and protect against sexually transmitted infections (STIs).

When used correctly every time you have sex, male condoms are 98% effective.

Condoms are a "barrier" method of contraception. They are made of very thin latex (rubber), polyurethane or polyisoprene and are designed to prevent pregnancy by stopping sperm from meeting an egg.

One of the main advantages of a Condom is when it is used correctly and consistently, is that they are a reliable method of preventing pregnancy and protecting both partners from STIs, including chlamydia, gonorrhoea and HIV.

Like anything there are also some disadvantages of Condoms. Some couples find that using condoms interrupts sex – to get around this, try to make using a condom part of foreplay.

Another disadvantage is that Condoms are very

strong but may split or tear if not used properly.

It is important to note once again that a Condom is the most reliable form of birth control as they are the only type of contraception that can both prevent pregnancy and protect against sexually transmitted infections (STIs).

The pill is a personal choice and it is important that you are aware of what the best type is for you.

What are some of the main risks and side effects of Hormonal Birth Control?

Cancer

Taking the combined pill will slightly increase the risk of breast cancer compared to people who are not taking it.

Even though we have seen many technological advancements over the years with hormonal contraceptives, a 2017 study showed that modern methods may carry the same cancer risks as the old high dose estrogen pills.

But it's important to remember that there are other things that have a bigger effect on breast cancer risk. For example, being overweight or obese increases the risk of breast cancer much more than taking the pill does.

When you stop taking the pill, your breast cancer risk stops increasing. About 10 years after stopping, a person's risk is no longer affected.

Blood clots

A serious risk of using birth control pills, especially combination pills, is an increased risk of blood clots. This can lead to:

- deep vein thrombosis (DVT)
- heart attack
- stroke
- pulmonary embolism

Overall, the risk of a blood clot from using any kind of birth control pill is low. According to the American Congress of Obstetricians and Gynaecologists, out of 10,000 women, fewer than 10 will develop a blood clot after taking a combination pill for a year. This risk is still lower than the risk of developing a blood clot during pregnancy and immediately after giving birth.

However, the risk of a blood clot from the pill is higher for certain women. This includes women who:

- are very overweight
- have high blood pressure
- are on bed rest for long periods

If any of these factors apply to you, talk with your doctor about the risks of using a birth control pill.

Depression

Depression and mood swings are commonly reported side effects of birth control pills.

Researchers have been unable to prove or disprove a link. The research is often conflicting.

A 2007 study showed that depression is the most common reason women stop using birth control pills. It also found women using combination birth control pills were "significantly more depressed" than a similar group of women not taking the pills. There may be a link to the fact that your natural hormones are not at play. Remember your progesterone is your calming hormone and the synthetic version is not as good as the real thing.

By contrast, a more recent study published in the AGO concluded that depression isn't a common side effect of birth control pills. This study maintained that the link between the two is unclear.

As the research is unclear and there is no definitive link it could be down to a variance in the pill chemical makeup of the pill itself.

Another very important factor is that there are currently a very high number of women with depression. Approximately 12 million in the US experience clinical depression each year. This could be down to timing or it could be down to consumption of the pill. It is very hard to say.

Even though the research is not definitive most pill manufacturers will list depression as a common side effect.

If you feel you may have depression it is important to know that there is support out there for you. You know your body better than anyone, don't forget that. If you're on birth control pills and experience depression symptoms for the first time, call your doctor. You should also call your doctor if previous depression symptoms worsen.

Hair Loss

Birth control pills can cause hair loss in women who are especially sensitive to the hormones in the pill or who have a family history of hormone-related hair loss.

Birth control pills cause the hair to move from the growing phase (also called anagen) to the resting phase (also called telogen) too soon and for too long.

Another factor that may come into play that a lot of women may think may not be applicable to them is the fact if baldness runs in your family, birth control pills can speed up the hair loss process.

Hair loss can also happen when you switch from one type of pill to another and can also happen during pregnancy.

Other hormonal birth control methods can also cause or worsen hair loss, including:

- hormone injections, such as Depo-Provera
- skin patches, such as Xulane
- progestin implants, such as Nexplanon
- vaginal rings, such as NuvaRing

So, what can you do to treat hair loss?

Hair loss caused by birth control pills is usually temporary. It should stop within a few months after your body gets used to the pill. Hair loss should also stop after you've been off of the pill for a while.

If the hair loss doesn't stop and you don't see regrowth, ask your doctor. There has been some evidence with Minoxidil 2% but it is best to check in with your doctor on this before you try anything. Please mention this with any discussion with your doctor on this topic.

As you consider birth control methods, think about your family history.

If hair loss runs in your family, look for pills that contain more estrogen than progestin. Because these pills can have other side effects, talk about the risks and the benefits with your doctor. If you have a strong family history of hair loss, a non-hormonal form of birth control may be a better choice.

Post Pill Acne

For women, birth control can be an option for treating acne because it regulates hormones that cause breakouts.

Birth control use and acne breakouts are linked, but in most cases it's for positive reasons. One of the main causes of acne is the presence of male hormones, particularly androgens. Androgens are found in both men and women. If you suffered with acne before going on the pill you may see it reappear after. This is due to it not getting to the root cause of why the acne occurred in the first place.

If you had acne when you were younger then it's likely that you were prescribed the combined oral contraceptive pill as this can be effective for managing acne especially around the time of your period. The progestogen-only pill or contraceptive implant, on the other hand, can sometimes make skin worse, so quitting the pill could actually make your skin better.

The reason that the combined pill is prescribed to manage acne is because taking both estrogen and progesterone lowers the number of androgens in your body. Androgens are a group of hormones which contain testosterone and these hormones stimulate the skin to produce sebum. A woman's ovaries and adrenal glands normally produce a low level of androgens but if you naturally have higher levels of androgens, then the pill suppresses them.

So, as we've already established, quitting the pill doesn't cause acne, it just removes the treatment that was controlling the problem.

When you stop taking the pill your ovaries try to return hormone levels back to normal, which can lead to an androgen rebound. Meaning the acne may reappear.

This means that the oil glands in your skin start producing more oil or sebum which triggers acne.

This sebum is often heavier than that which was produced when you were on the pill. This sebum then gets stuck in the pores and blocks them causing blackheads behind which bacteria grows, leading to more severe forms of pimples such as cysts and pustules.

There are other reasons why your skin flares up after quitting the pill. Firstly, it's well documented that the pill depletes many of the nutrients that your skin needs to stay healthy.

When you quit the pill your zinc levels will be depleted which also contributes to acne and breakouts. This is because Zinc helps to regulate testosterone, it kills the bacteria on the skin that causes acne, and it reduces keratin production that blocks pores. So, less zinc = more breakouts.

Secondly, you might experience breakouts because taking the pill consistently also affects your gut flora which can cause inflammation in your skin. So, you'll need to take care of yourself inside and out to manage your post-pill acne.

How long does post-pill acne last?

It's hard to say and it really varies from person to person. But post pill acne typically peaks around 3-6 months after ditching the birth control pill and it can take months to treat. It won't go away on its own, so treating your post-pill acne will require sticking to a consistent skincare routine for a number of months.

What can you do to manage my post-pill acne?

Well, the first thing you can do is to accept that it's not your fault

Some treatments that may work include:

- Reducing dairy if you feel you break out. Currently there is no link between dairy and acne. It is normally the danger in the dose. This is very people dependent so please keep an eye on this.
- Look at digestive issues like IBS and SIBO
- Look into the possibility of histamine intolerance
- Zinc
- Skincare routine
- Stress management
- Berberine. **Please note** that berberine is not safe for long term use and should be taken for no longer than 8 weeks. If you have gut issues, please be mindful that this can aggravate the problems.
- DIM (diindolylmethane)

Although post-pill acne can be difficult to manage and can really knock your confidence, there are lots of things you can do to manage it. Remember the pill is only masking the symptoms so it will not be the long-term answer. If you are still struggling with acne making an appointment with your doctor or a dermatologist could be the next move.

Post Pill PMS

When you stop the pill, you may find that you get a new symptom that you may not have had before or one that has come back with a vengeance and that is PMS. The reason for this is due to having cycles for the first time in a very long time or ever. The cycles that you were having before were "pill cycles" and were due to synthetic hormones being pumped into the body. While the real cycle "post pill cycles") are your naturally occurring hormones and it can take time to apart to this natural up and down.

The question that may come into your mind if this is you is "If I can do without PMS why do I need to have a real period?"

The answer is that your real hormones are much better for your health. Check out the PMS chapter of the book for tips to manage this.

Post Pill Amenorrhea & Post Pill PCOS

If you have come off the pill and you haven't got your cycle back yet, you need to ask a very important question "what was your cycle like before?"

If you don't have a period for several months, you may have what's known as post-pill amenorrhea. The pill prevents your body from making hormones involved in ovulation and menstruation. When you stop taking the pill, it can take some time for your body to start producing these hormones again.

If your cycle was irregular before, then there was an issue then, and the pill is simply masking the issue. You must get to the root cause of why this was happening if you want your body to work for you. Band aid over a broken leg comes to mind.
If your cycle was regular before and now, they are irregular after coming off the pill then you have post pill PCOS or post pill Amenorrhea. Please check out the PCOS chapter for more information on post pill PCOS and how to treat it.

Menstrual periods typically resume within three months after you stop taking the pill. But if you took the pill to regulate your menstrual cycles, it may take several months before your period comes back. Please check out the chapters on these two topics later on in the book for more information.

If you don't have a period within three months, take a pregnancy test to make sure you're not pregnant and then see your doctor.

If you are trying or have an active sex life the sex section below could be really helpful.

Does the pill affect sex drive?

This is a hard question to answer.

Studying sex, libido (sex drive), and sexual pleasure is complicated. Your sex drive and sexual pleasure are impacted by your physiology, psychology, societal expectations and the interactions between these.

In addition, we still don't have a great understanding of the female sexual anatomy or female orgasm. The likes of Jenny Keane (@hellojennykeane) are doing incredible work in Ireland on how to make your body work for you and to educate women and their partners on sex and orgasms.

Here's what the research says about each type of birth control

<u>Combined hormonal contraceptives and sex</u>

This type of birth control includes the combined-hormone pill (i.e., oral contraceptives or the pill), the vaginal ring, and the hormonal patch. These forms of birth control contain a form of estrogen and a progestin (a synthetic progesterone). CHC works by suppressing ovulation and thickening cervical mucus.

Studies into the effect of combined pills on sexual functioning do not all agree with one another. Most studies have found no impact or improved sexual functioning among users of the pill.

In a 2013 review of studies published since the 1970s on the pill and sexual function, researchers found that more than 6 in 10 people using the pill had no changes in libido, more than 2 in 10 had an increase in libido, and about 1 in 10 did report a decrease in libido.

Different formulations (chemical make-ups) and the varying number of days a person takes a hormone-pill vs no pill or a placebo-pill, may impact sexual functioning. Pill regimens that have more hormone-containing pill days than the common 21-hormone/7-placebo pills may be more likely to improve sexual functioning.

Lower amounts of estrogen may cause more changes to sex drive than higher amounts (this is called a dose-response relationship).
In the 2013 study, all people using pills with the smallest dose of estrogen available (15 micrograms), reported having a decreased libido, while people using pills with higher doses of estrogen reported mostly no change or an increase in libido. The number of people using low-dose pills was small—only 140 people—so it's difficult to say if these results are applicable to everyone.

Some studies have looked at more than just libido.

A 2016 randomized control trial examined how people using one formulation of the pill differed, sexually, from people using a placebo (i.e. a pill that contains no drug) in seven areas of sexual function. They found that people in the pill group were more likely to report decreased sexual desire, arousal, and pleasure.

However, decreased arousal and desire did not seem to mean less sex, or less good sex. Both groups reported about the same number of "satisfying sexual episodes" and the same scores for questions about orgasm.

One-way CHCs may negatively impact sex drive is by lowering the level of testosterone in the body.

Lower testosterone is thought to decrease sex drive, but the relationship between testosterone and sex drive is not well understood. People with abnormally high levels of testosterone, such as people with PCOS, don't necessarily have higher libido; however, people with consistently low libidos sometimes benefit from testosterone supplementation.

In a 2016 randomized trial, researchers found that people using the pill had lower testosterone levels than they did at the beginning of the study, and lower levels than the placebo group at follow-up. Despite this difference, testosterone levels were not associated with any differences in sexual function, suggesting that the lower testosterone may not be the cause for the reported difference.

The ring and the patch

The hormonal vaginal ring and patch are less studied than the pill. So please take this into account when reading the information below.

One review study found that users of the ring were three times more likely to report vaginal wetness and less likely to report vaginal dryness, as opposed to people using the pill. Both pill and ring users reported improved sexual functioning, including higher scores on sexual pleasure and orgasm, as compared to people using non-hormonal methods.

In a randomized control trial where people were assigned to the combined pill or the ring, both pill and ring users reported higher sexual functioning at

3 and 6 months.

Certain types of CHCs, extended use (packs that have 24-day hormone pills), and continuous use (packs that have people using hormone-containing pills for a few months) can also reduce the frequency of menstrual migraines and negative premenstrual symptoms, which may improve a person's mood and overall sex life.

Progestin-only contraceptives and sex

The pill (e.g., "mini pill")

Progestin-only pills are pills that only contain progestin (so they don't contain estrogen). They work primarily by thickening cervical mucus.

There are very few studies that have looked at sexual function among progestin-only users. In a study where participants used combined pills, progestin-only pills, and the vaginal ring for 3 months each, people reported higher sexual interest during the 3 months that they used the vaginal ring as compared to either pill type.

Researchers also found that the types of birth control affected participants' testosterone levels. This relationship was modified by genetics, specifically the sensitivity of androgen receptors, or the proteins on cells that "read" androgens, in each participant (testosterone is a type of androgen).

In a study that included participants from Scotland and the Philippines, the progestin-only pill had no impact on sexual interest or activity at four months in comparison to a placebo.

Interestingly, the combined pill had a negative impact on sex for participants from Scotland, but not for participants from the Philippines, suggesting that physiology and/or socio-cultural experiences may impact birth control acceptability.

Injection (Progestin-Only)

Progestin-only injection, sometimes better known by the brand names Depo-Provera/DMPA and Noristerat, is a form of contraception that only contains a progestin.

There is not much research on the impact of injectable contraception on sex drive.

One study in the United States found that after six months of use, people using DMPA were 2 to 3 times more likely to report that they were "lacking interest in sex" than people using the copper IUD, which does not contain hormones.

In a study conducted in Kenya, about 1 in 10 people using DMPA reported "reduced libido" during 6 months of use and 2 out of 15 people who stopped using DMPA reported reduced libido.

DMPA doesn't necessarily have a negative effect on everyone, though.

In the Kenya study, there was no average change in "sexual interest" or "arousal", and the average scores for "enjoyment" and "orgasm" increased.

Another study among adolescents aged 14-17 found no differences in reported sexual interest between users of DMPA, users of combined pills, and people who didn't use hormonal methods. A study among adults reached similar conclusions.

One benefit of the shot that might improve a person's sex life is that it doesn't require taking a pill every day or using a condom to prevent pregnancy—someone only needs to worry about birth control method every 8 to 12 weeks. The shot can also reduce menstrual bleeding and migraines, which may increase the number of days a person wants to have sex.

Implant (e.g., Nexplanon)

The contraceptive implant (e.g., Implanon, Nexplanon) is a device that contains only progestin.

Less than 1 in 20 people using the implant report a decrease in libido, though estimates vary. This is a very small sample of people so more research is needed.
In one study, users of the implant were more likely to report that they lacked interest in sex as compared to users of the copper IUD. Despite this, few people discontinue using the implant due to lost libido.

One study reported improved overall sexual functioning and improved sexual satisfaction after 3 and 6 months with the implant. This suggests that the implant may negatively impact a small number of users' sex lives, but for the majority it either improves or does not change their sex lives.

The implant may improve someone's sex life by reducing the stress of worrying about unintended pregnancies.

Hormonal and Copper IUDs

There are two types of IUDs: hormonal and copper. The hormonal IUDs (e.g. Mirena, Kylena, and Lilleta).

In general, hormonal and copper IUDs users report that their method of birth control has no impact on or improves their sexual satisfaction.

One study found that 9 out of 10 people using either type of IUD had no change in libido and 3 out of 10 reported increased sexual spontaneity.

The hormonal IUD has also been associated with more sexual desire, decreased sexual pain, and lower levels of sexual dysfunction, compared to function before using the IUD, or compared with people not using contraception.

Like the implant and the shot, IUDs are a great choice for people who don't want to think about their birth control every day. IUDs are also one of the most effective forms of birth control. Although hormonal IUD users may initially experience prolonged or abnormal bleeding, the hormonal IUD tends to decrease menstrual bleeding and menstrual pain after a few months of use, which may improve a person's sexual experience.

What to do if you think your birth control is negatively affecting your sex life

Choosing a birth control method isn't a lifelong commitment. Even if you decide to use the implant or an IUD, you can always have them removed before they expire.

If you're otherwise happy with your method, you may want to consider if other things going on in your life, such as stress or your relationship with your partner, may be causing your changes in sexual function as opposed to your birth control.

If you're new to starting a method, you could consider waiting a few months to see if your body adjusts to your new method of birth control. However, it's 100% your decision as to when to stop using a method. You don't have to wait to change methods if you don't want to.

Whether you're using birth control or not, you can use apps like Natural Cycles, Clue, Kindara or even a notebook to track both your sexual frequency and sex drive. Tracking can help you make an informed decision about starting, stopping, or switching methods of birth control. This is one of the most important things you can do for your body is understand how it works for you.

FAQ

There are many questions that come with the pill and here are some of the most common ones I come across on a regular basis.

Do I get a "real" period on the contraceptive pill?

Nope. The bleeding you get when you're on the pill is not the same as a menstrual period.
Your period on the pill is technically called withdrawal bleeding, referring to the withdrawal of hormones in your pill, and in your body. The drop in hormone levels causes the lining of your uterus (the endometrium) to shed. This bleeding may be slightly different than the period you had before taking the pill. It also may change over time while taking the pill.

What exactly is happening to my body? Do I ovulate on the contraceptive pill?

No. If you take your pill consistently and correctly, you shouldn't ovulate. This is the primary way the pill prevents pregnancy. In a usual (no-pill) cycle, the body's natural reproductive hormones fluctuate up and down, taking your body through a process of preparing an egg for release, releasing that egg, and preparing your uterus to accept a potentially fertilized egg.

The hormones in the contraceptive pill stop and prevent your ovaries from preparing and releasing eggs. They stop the usual hormonal "cycling", including ovulation, the typical growth of the endometrium, and the natural period.

Why is my bleeding different on the contraceptive pill?

The contraceptive pill prevents the lining of your uterus (your endometrium) from growing thicker, as it would in a typical menstrual cycle. It also prevents ovulation and the typical cycling of reproductive hormones. When you have withdrawal bleeding, the bleeding tends to be lighter than normal menstrual bleeding.

It's also possible to have no withdrawal bleeding or only spotting during the days you take inactive pills (or no pills). This is more common for people taking higher doses of estrogen, or a pill with a shorter (or no) hormone-free interval (most pill packs have seven placebo pills but check your pack's box and info sheet if you're not sure or talk to your healthcare provider.)

What kind of bleeding is considered normal while on the contraceptive pill?

- Unexpected spotting for the first few months while taking a new pill (talk to your healthcare provider if it's still happening after 3 months)
- Withdrawal bleeding that is lighter, or shorter than your period before you were taking the pill
- Withdrawal bleeding that changes slightly over time while on the pill

- Having little or no bleeding during your placebo week after taking your pills correctly

I'm having unexpected bleeding on the contraceptive pill, what do I do?

Spotting can happen outside of your usual withdrawal bleed time. This is called breakthrough bleeding. It doesn't mean your pill isn't working, but it can be frustrating to deal with. Up to 1 in 5 people experience breakthrough bleeding when first taking the contraceptive pill.

It is not usually a cause for concern and will often stop after a few weeks or months. Others will need to try a different pill brand, with different levels of hormones. Many experts recommend choosing a pill with the lowest dose of estrogen (ethinylestradiol/EE), and only changing to a higher dose if breakthrough bleeding is a persistent problem.

Spotting can also be caused by missed pills, as the drop in hormone levels can cause a small amount of withdrawal bleeding.

Will I gain weight on the pill?

This is a common thought. But studies have shown that the effect of the birth control pill on weight is small — if it exists at all.

The truth is there is a very real possibility that women differ in their exposure to gain weight in response to the use of hormonal BC (BC = birth control). Women tend to report different physical, emotional and other side effects from different types of BC, and it would seem reasonable to assume that the metabolic effects could also differ.

There is some indication that women already carrying more body fat are more likely to gain fat from BC so there may be an interaction here with either the pre-existing physiology or lifestyle factors such as diet or activity.

Generally, with age, there is a gain in body weight, and some studies find that the weight gain that occurs with hormonal BC is about the same as what is seen in women using non-hormonal BC or nothing at all.

Research would also show that black women are more prone to weight gain with BC.

Hormonal BC may be getting blamed for what is primarily nothing more than age or lifestyle-related weight gain. The change in body composition can't be ignored.

Body composition decreasing or weight gain increasing is not ideal for anyone but it appears that most forms of BC have minimal impact on body composition decreasing or weight increasing.

Even in the absence of true or even significant weight gain a worsening of body composition is never good and it looks the overall effect of most forms of BC on body weight appears to be mild at best.

Sorry, but we cannot really blame the pill for weight gain.

If you are looking for more information on this please look into Lyle McDonalds work in particular, the Women's Book Vol 1: A guide to Nutrition, Fat loss and Muscle Gain. If you are a coach or trainer and you want a book to learn about how to coach women this book alongside the work by Dr. Stacy Sims is revolutionary.

If you plan to have a baby, how soon after stopping birth control pills can you conceive?

Usually, ovulation begins again a few weeks after stopping birth control pills.

As soon as you ovulate again, you can get pregnant. If this happens during your first cycle off the pill, you may not have a period at all. Take a pregnancy test if you've had unprotected sex and your period hasn't returned.

Is there an advantage to waiting a few months after stopping the pill before trying to conceive?

Conceiving immediately after stopping the pill does not increase your risk of miscarriage or harm to the foetus. The hormones in birth control pills don't remain in your system.

Usually, periods start again a few weeks after stopping the pill. However, if your periods were infrequent before you started taking the pill, they will likely be that way again after you stop taking the pill. It may take a couple of months before you return to regular ovulation cycles.

After stopping the pill, if you're not ready to conceive, consider using a backup form of birth control.

What happens if I take birth control pills while pregnant?

Don't worry if you kept taking your birth control pill because you didn't know you were pregnant.

Despite years of this accident happening, there's very little evidence that exposure to the hormones in birth control pills causes birth defects. Once you learn that you're pregnant, stop taking the birth control pill.

Can I use several birth control pills at once for emergency contraception?

It's possible to use standard estrogen-progestin birth control pills for emergency contraception, but check with your doctor for the proper dose and timing of the pills.

Certain types of pills are specifically designed to keep you from becoming pregnant if you've had unprotected sex. These medications are sometimes referred to as the morning-after pill.

Morning-after pills contain either levonorgestrel (Plan B One-Step, EContra One-Step, others) or ulipristal acetate (ella, Logilia).

Levonorgestrel pills are available over-the-counter to anyone of any age. Levonorgestrel pills work best when used as soon as possible — and within three days — after unprotected sex.

Ulipristal acetate is a non-hormonal medication available only by prescription. This medication is taken as a single dose within five days after unprotected sex.

A copper intrauterine device (IUD) or an IUD containing 52 milligrams of levonorgestrel may also be used for emergency contraception. Ideally, these IUDs should be placed by your doctor within five days of unprotected intercourse.

Does how much you weigh reduce the effectiveness of emergency birth control pills?

If you are considered obese with a body mass index (BMI) of 30 or more, emergency contraception may not be as effective — especially if you use levonorgestrel. You could still become pregnant after using levonorgestrel for emergency contraception. BMI is not as much of a concern when using ulipristal. Use of an IUD for emergency birth control is not affected by body weight.

I have taken birth control pills for years and want to stop. Can I stop at any time or should I finish my current pill packet?

In terms of your overall health, it makes little

difference when you stop taking the pill. When you finally do stop the pill, you can expect some bleeding, which may change the rhythm of your menstrual cycle. But you can stop at any time.

Can I get pregnant during the week of inactive pills?

Taking the inactive pills doesn't put you at higher risk of unintended pregnancy. If you're taking birth control pills exactly as directed, they're about 99% effective at preventing pregnancy.

But if you miss a pill — or several pills — during a cycle, you might be at higher risk of unintended pregnancy during that cycle. To be safe, use a backup form of contraception, such as a condom, especially if you miss several pills during a cycle.

How do birth control pills affect cancer risk?

Most data show that birth control pills don't increase your overall risk of cancer.

Scientific evidence suggests using birth control pills for longer periods of time increases your risk of some cancers, such as cervical cancer, but the risk declines after stopping use of birth control pills.

Regarding breast cancer risk, the results are mixed. Some studies show a link between birth control pill use and a slight increase in breast cancer risk, but the risk is very low. Other studies have shown no significant increase in breast cancer risk. Risk appears to decrease over time after discontinuing birth control pills. If you have a family history of breast cancer, birth control use does not appear to increase the risk.

The birth control pill may decrease your risk of other types of cancer, including ovarian cancer, endometrial cancer and colon cancer — and this benefit may persist for years after you stop the pill.

Do birth control pills affect cholesterol levels?

Birth control pills can affect your cholesterol levels. How much of an effect depends on the type of pill you're taking and what concentration of estrogen or progestin it contains. Birth control pills with more estrogen can have a slightly beneficial overall effect on your cholesterol levels. In general, though, the changes aren't significant and don't affect your overall health.

Do birth control pills affect blood pressure?

Birth control pills may slightly increase your blood pressure. If you take birth control pills, have your blood pressure checked regularly. If you already have high blood pressure, talk with your doctor about whether you should consider another form of birth control.

What is the risk of blood clots when taking birth control pills?

The estrogen contained in combination hormone birth control pills and in the ring or patch is not recommended if you have a history of blood clots — venous thromboembolism (VTE) — or if you are at high risk of blood clots. A progestin-only form of contraception — such as the mini pill or an implant — an IUD or a barrier method is a better choice. Progestin or progesterone also can increase the risk of blood clots, but the risk is less than with estrogen.

Can antibiotics decrease the effectiveness of birth control pills?

Antibiotics do not interfere with the effectiveness of birth control pills — except in the case of one antibiotic, rifampin (Rimactane). Rifampin does decrease the effectiveness of birth control pills in preventing ovulation, but this antibiotic isn't widely used today.

Conclusion

Freedom off the pill

The pill is such a personal choice so please remember this. When you come off the pill it allows you to understand your body like never before and allows you to become in tune with it. I am neither before or against the pill. I am prochoice.

It serves a purpose (managing heavy flow etc, managing endometriosis to name but a few) but if your goal is overall health long term it may be an option to link in with your doctor and chat through your options alongside your partner or family.

As you can see from the above sections hormonal

birth control has shown links to depression, hair loss, nutrient deficiencies and some impact on sex drive.

If you are looking for the best option for birth control, if possible, please choose a non-hormonal birth control option, like the non-hormonal IUD, or even ask your partner to wear a condom. Remember it takes two to tango.

Hormonal birth control can also cause high blood pressure, nutrient deficiency and some reduced thyroid function, reduction in bone health and issues with digestion and gut health.

There are many benefits with coming off the pill, the main one being regular cycles. But like anything there can be side effects of going off the pill and these include Post-Pill Acne, PMS and Amenorrhea (or lack of a cycle).

Chapter 4 - Hypothalamic Amenorrhea (HA)

The next few chapters are going to go through the various conditions and cycle issues that women may face during their lifetime including HA, PCOS, Endometriosis, Thyroid, Perimenopause, Menopause and Pregnancy.

The first one of these that we are going to look at is Hypothalamic Amenorrhea or HA for short hand. So, where you see the letters HA it means Hypothalamic Amenorrhea.

What is HA?

Hypothalamic Amenorrhea is defined as the lack of a menstrual cycle period of more than six months when no medical diagnosis can be found. The last part of this sentence is very important.

The no medical diagnosis means your doctor should have ruled out other conditions such as thyroid disease, celiac disease, PCOS, high prolactin and others.

There are two main types of Amenorrhea. Those who haven't begun to menstruate by age 16 may have Primary Amenorrhea. The term also applies to abnormalities in the reproductive tract that prevent menstrual bleeding. Primary Amenorrhea can result from structural problems with your sex organs. It may be a sign of underdeveloped or malfunctioning ovaries.

Issues with your pituitary or thyroid glands can result

in Secondary Amenorrhea. When working properly, these glands produce the hormones needed for menstruation.

If you miss your monthly period for 3 straight months after having regular cycles for the previous 9 months, you may have Secondary Amenorrhea. This type of Amenorrhea is more common.

It is important to look at another very important factor that could cause the lack of a cycle, and that is coming off the Pill (also known as Post-Pill Amenorrhea). Please talk to your medical professional about this. If they suggest going back on the pill this is not the answer. This is like sticking a band aid on a broken arm and hope it solves the issue.

Please be aware that it's normal not to have a period during pregnancy or after menopause. But if you miss periods at other times, it may be a symptom of an underlying medical issue.

The role of Hypothalamus

If there is no medical reason for your lack of periods, then it's because your hypothalamus (the control centre for your hormones) has decided that you should not ovulate.

If the Hypothalamus has decided that it doesn't want you to ovulate then it means it has gone into safety mode and is trying to protect you from outside stressors.

Three of the main factors are that you are very stressed or that you are under-eating to fuel your body or you are over exercising.

If the Hypothalamus feels that it is in danger it will shut off ovulation to protect you against having a baby. The Hypothalamus will dial down the hormones that promote reproduction until the environment is safe to do so. The body is a lot smarter than we give it credit for.
It's important to note that Hypothalamic Amenorrhea is not a disorder and that is a normal response to under eating or stress.

What are the main risk factors for HA?

HA results in estrogen deficiency and the cessation of the menstrual cycle in young premenopausal women. This, in turn, has significant effects on the body's cardiac, skeletal, psychological, and reproductive system. These effects can mimic menopause and all the physical and psychological changes that it works on the body.

Short term consequences of amenorrhea include low estrogen and the accompanying hair thinning or loss, brittle nails, skin problems, low libido, and vagina dryness.

One difficulty is that many women with HA, due to lack of symptoms, often feel quite well. Thus, they may be reluctant to seek treatment.

Longer-term consequences include higher cardiovascular disease risk and threatened bone health. Low estrogen suppresses bone production, which can lead to bone loss, osteopenia (loss of bone calcium), and increased risk of fractures.

Amenorrhea can cause bone loss in as little as six months. HA is also implicated in increasing depression and anxiety. HA can cause an absence of ovulation and infertility during a woman's peak reproductive years.

My point is that HA is so much more than a missing period and subtle symptoms should not be ignored. If your period has gone missing there is nothing "normal" about that.

Don't let the problem go on for longer than it needs to. Getting help and support is the first and most important step in making a full recovery!

Because the good news is that getting your period back naturally is completely possible!

Treating amenorrhea

Your doctor's recommended treatment plan for Amenorrhea will depend on its underlying cause.

If it's linked to obesity, your doctor will likely recommend a weight loss program. If extreme weight loss or excessive exercising is the reason, they'll encourage you to gain weight or exercise less.

To help you manage your mental health, your doctor

may also prescribe therapy, medications, or other treatments.

To treat issues with your thyroid gland, your doctor may prescribe medications like hormone replacements or recommend surgery.

For ovarian cancer, your doctor may recommend a combination of medications, radiation therapy, and chemotherapy.

Medication or surgery to treat other conditions that can cause Amenorrhea are also options.
If your doctor recommends going on contraception, please get a second opinion as this will only start an artificial bleed and not a real one.

This happens way too often and shows a lack of duty of care towards the woman in question. The pill is not the solution!

The Pill is not the solution

Unfortunately, when suffering from HA, many women are prescribed the pill long before they are given the recommendation to change their lifestyle. The pill is not a solution to Hypothalamic Amenorrhea, it's a band-aid prescription that masks the problem.

With the pill, it is an estrogen replacement that will provide a fake bleed, it does not solve the underlying problem or help the resumption of normal natural hormone activity. The underlying HA still needs to be addressed and birth control pills may only mask the problem.

If you're getting your period back due to being on the pill but you're still under-eating and over-exercising...the problem has not been solved. Your bones are still getting weaker (another thing the pill doesn't protect!) and your body is still crying out for help.

Changing your lifestyle is essential to recovery – there honestly is no other solution.

I know lifestyle changes are scary and daunting, but I promise you, I've helped lots of clients overcome HA.

Relying on the pill to get your cycle back is like relying on a potato to start a car. It won't end too well.

Preventing amenorrhea

Two of the main factors (if it is not an underlying medical issue) are stress and under-eating/over-exercising.

For a woman to get her period she needs to be fully nourished in every respect. This means getting enough calories (fuel) and getting enough carbohydrates and fats into their body. Unfortunately, these two foods have a lot of stigma and fear around them but if you are looking to get your cycle back it is so important that you fuel yourself correctly.

Carbohydrates are like the key that starts the engine when it comes to your cycle and promotes healthy ovulation. They also lead to increased insulin, which signals energy availability to the hypothalamus for production of GnRH and the cascade of reproductive hormones that follow including increased FSH and LH.

Please note that under-eating carbohydrates can impair hypothalamic signalling and cause amenorrhea - even when you are getting enough calories. The power of carbohydrates is not to be downplayed at all and there is zero need to fear them.

The role of fats cannot be downplayed either. Fat plays a role in hormone production. Sex hormones (such as estrogen, progesterone and testosterone) are made from cholesterol. If fat and cholesterol are cut out of the diet, a steady supply of estrogen isn't produced, causing symptoms of low estrogen as seen in HA.

Let's not forget about Protein. Eating sufficient protein is important as hormones are made from protein and fat. Amino acids (the building blocks of protein) are also used for lots of other physiological processes in the body.

Managing Psychological Stress

Managing stress is a major factor on the body. If the body is very stressed the Hypothalamus can go into safety mode and turn off ovulation to protect the body.

Some of these techniques can help:

- Therapy/CBT
- Mindfulness or Meditation
- Work on reducing perfectionism
- Self-compassion
- Set and communicate Boundaries

Please talk to your doctor about any concerns you have about your menstrual cycle. It is imperative that when you are with your doctor that you get a full hormone screen. This will allow you to see what exactly is going on. Think of it like a mechanic trying to work on a car, they need to look under the hood first in order to understand what is going on.

If your medical professional makes this difficult, please make sure to be strong on this as you have the right to understand how your body works for you. If they refuse, please find another medical professional.

The importance of regular meals

Intermittent fasting, otherwise known as time restricted feeding, is currently one of the world's most popular health and fitness trends where you alternate between periods of feeding and fasting.

Intermittent fasting is an eating pattern where you cycle between periods of eating and fasting. The most popular form of intermittent fasting is known as the 16/8 method. This is when you're technically fasting for 16 hours every day, and restricting you're eating to an 8-hour eating window.

It's touted for many health benefits, but are these benefits evidence-based and do they apply the same to men as they do women???

Looking at the research, the answer is no. Mostly because the research to date is mostly on rats, not humans.

And a couple of those studies have found that intermittent fasting can make female rats emaciated, masculinized, infertile and cause them to miss cycles.

Anecdotal evidence from many women I've worked with and around the fitness space also reaffirm this with missing cycles starting during Intermittent Fasting. More evidence is needed on this and if you feel good through Intermittent fasting please continue. But if you are using Intermittent Fasting and you are having issues with your cycle then this is where things may need to be looked at.

Regardless of the health benefits, if your approach to nutrition and eating causes you to lose your period, it's unhealthy.

During recovery from HA it's really important to break these mindsets around meal timing and delayed eating because consistent intake of food throughout the day is absolutely critical for you to get your period back.

By eating constantly throughout the day, you have a greater chance of hitting that minimum of fuelling your body for recovery. Additionally, frequent eating prevents within day energy deficits which is known to cause a longer time to period recovery.

So, what's the best way to eat if you're trying to get your period back?

A solid 3 meals and 3 snacks per day is a great place to start. You may also need more eating occasions depending on your life and circumstances.

Recovery requires eating enough—not only to adequately fuel current energy needs but to also to make up for the history of under-fuelling. For most women with HA, eating a greater variety of foods, from all macronutrient groups including fats and starches, seems to stimulate more hormone production.

Please try to remove calorie counting from your routine if it is something that is causing a trigger. If you are coming from a background of an eating disorder, please do talk to a mental health professional or your medical provider.

Are 2,500 calories the magic number?

With HA recovery there is a general recommendation of at least 2,500 calories for period recovery, but where does this come from and is it the amount you need?

The truth is 2,500 calories isn't a magic number!

You may need a different amount for this for recovery.

The basis for this number is from Dr. Nicola Rinaldi's book "No period, Now What?" and is actually a general recommendation based on a study in 2007 by Anne Loucks and her colleagues where they looked at endurance athletes' dietary requirements to be what they termed "energy replete" and calculated this to be at 45 calories per kilo of fat-free body mass. But this is a generic number and no one on this planet is generic.

How much do you need to eat will need depend on a variety of factors including?

- Your health history
- Your height and starting weight
- Your level of exercise
- Yor age
- And many more

The more repair and restore work your body have to do, the more energy you will require. The more active you are, the more your body needs. If you are still in a growth period of life it's likely you need a lot more e.g. puberty.

The biggest factor though is you are a human, you are not a robot and the amount of food you need each day varies day to day. Therefore 2,500 calories are not the secret and aiming to fuel yourself more will help you in the long run.

Should you count calories during HA recovery?

This is such a common question that is asked and my general recommendation is "NO", and here is why:

- This is the time to be learning about adequate portion sizes, balanced meals and not hitting a perfect macro split.
- Many people use calories to determine if a food or meal is "allowed" when this is the time to be breaking away from those rules.
- Your hunger levels vary and honouring that may be more difficult if you don't think you can go above a certain number of calories each day.
- It takes up a lot of time/headspace to do this each day.
- It creates dependency and then there is anxiety related towards letting it go because of fear of under eating.

A health professional will be able to teach you adequate portion sizes, meal and snack ideas for your needs without counting.

In addition to reversing low energy availability, it also about addressing your:

- Overall health and lifestyle
- Relationship with food and exercise
- Stress Levels
- Body Image
- Mindset

Remember HA recovery is more than calories.

How to increase your calorie intake in recovery?

One of the things I discuss with clients as they move into recovery is the necessity of nourishing their body adequately so they can weight restore if necessary and reverse low energy availability to get their period back.

I like to use the analogy of a mobile phone. You make sure that you charge that fully at night so why not do that for your own body?

A big problem is that many of the clients I work with often underestimate just how much energy it takes to repair and restore their body so that all systems function optimally again and they have extra energy and vitality in their day to day lives.

Added to this is the fact that diet culture often warps our perception of what a normal portion is and also what kinds of foods we should be eating.

This can make eating and decisions around food feel so much harder than it needs to be, so let's break down a few simple ways to increase your calorie intake:

> 1. Regular Meals - Start out by increasing eating occasions up to 3 meals and 3 snacks as a minimum. Eating every 2-3 hours is a good guide to provide your body with consistent nutrition and help keep your blood sugar levels stable.

2. Adequacy - Once you've got those eating occasions down, then the focus is on ensuring you are including all food groups and in adequate amounts for your body and recovery goals. Typically, you start with safer foods here and then work towards tackling foods you feel less comfortable with alongside breaking down food rules.

3. Volume vs. Density - Overfilling on low-calorie high-volume foods can lead to lots of digestive distress, so here we focus on providing the body with more nourishing options that will give the body nutrition it needs. This also naturally helps us veer away from low calorie and diet products.

4. Honouring Hunger - As you begin to eat more you may feel quite full initially, but as your metabolism and body work to restore your hunger levels will return. Responding to these will help build trust in your body and support the physical process of recovery at the same time.

The role of weight gain in HA recovery

You may not want to gain weight, thinking that you already feel healthy. However, if you are not menstruating due to HA, your body disagrees with you.

With the increased calories that your body is thanking you for, your weight may start to increase. You may be pleasantly surprised to see your cycles resume. Although healthy body weights vary greatly, most women with HA need to obtain a BMI of 22 to 23 or even higher to resume menses, but some may need more.

This can be a massive adjustment for some and understandably so. I would aim to try to include some of these tips if you are trying to gain weight:

1. Remove the scales if it is triggering you
2. Work with a dietitian or a mental health professional
3. Have a support network
4. Remove any clothes that you don't feel are adding to your life
5. Edit your social media feed to remove any fitness or any accounts that trigger you
6. Be patient

How long will it take to get your period back after committing to HA recovery?

The timing question is one that I get all too often and I always joke that my crystal ball is broken because it's impossible to predict when a period will return.

But to help ease your mind I'm answering some of the most common questions surrounding time to recovery.

According to surveys done by Dr. Nicola Rinaldi from No Period Now What, the median time is 3 months (so 50% get their first period before this time, and 50% get it after this time). So, the average length of time is 5.4 months but it can take others longer and sometimes it can take a shorter time period.

But I need to stress that everyone's timeline is different and you need to be patient!
The most critical factor for your success will be to change your mind set about what being healthy truly means so that changing your lifestyle in terms of food and exercise feels easier. Because consistency and patience are key.

How long YOUR body needs to feel safe is highly individual, but I promise with the implementation of a good recovery plan you will get there!

Does length of time without a period impact how long it will take to recover from hypothalamic amenorrhea?

In short, no it doesn't. You could be without a period for 3 months or 10 years and it could take the same amount of time.

What factors influence recovery time?

The three factors that play the biggest role are how quickly you optimise your energy availability through eating more, exercising less and managing your stress.

If you need to gain a significant amount of weight to reach a fertile BMI then it could take you a bit longer so be patient. If you are struggling with this then please link with a professional to help guide you along the way.

Exercise during HA recovery

HA recovery is about recovery and one of the big things that will be needed to be looked at will be reducing exercise. As this will ultimately reduce the energy expended by the body and can take stress off the body. People don't realise that exercise is a stressor on the body.

Advised exercise

- Gentle or restorative yoga
- Mat Pilates
- Modified weight training (x3 sessions max a week)
- Mindful walking
- Rehabilitative exercises
- No fasted training
- No training to failure

Exercise to be mindful of

- CrossFit - the body is under a huge amount of stress during this form of exercise
- HIIT style training
- Power Yoga
- Heavy Weight Training
- Running
- Long Duration cardio (including treadmills, stair masters etc)

If you are sore, have low energy, feel faint some

alongside not fuelling yourself then it's so important that you look at the form of exercise and ask yourself "*Is this the best thing I can be doing to aid my HA recovery?*"

Supplementation

HA is generally reversible and predictive factors seem to include a higher basal BMI and lower serum cortisol levels (stress hormone). It is so important that you try to restore your cycle through reduced exercise, readied stress and an increase in calories before looking to go down the supplementation route.

There are currently no supplements with strong evidence to support restoration alone.

Some supplements that may have potential:

- Vitex (Agnus Castus)
- Calcium is essential for strong bones and because HA causes bone loss we are trying to ensure we give your body the best chance at protecting bone mass and building some back once your period returns!
- Iron is also very important as the body transports oxygen via haemoglobin which we get from iron, without enough we start to feel breathless and fatigued. Optimising these levels before your period starts will ensure you don't lose too much through your monthly menstrual cycle which can happen if you have heavy periods

- Vitamin D (the sunshine vitamin) helps with calcium absorption and bone health. Get your daily dose or consider a supplement if deficient, 1000iu for bone health.
- Acetyl-l- carnitine may have potential at 2g per day

Others that require more research include:
- Myo Inositol

Please do not take these all in one go. Please consult with a Nutritionist or a Dietitian to guide you on what the best protocol for you is. Supplements are there to aid your diet and lifestyle, they do not work in isolation.

I have seen great results with Vitex when working with clients (alongside ensuring adequate rest, food and stress management). Please do not take Vitex if you are pregnant, breastfeeding or on any medication for mental health.

Conclusion

While missing a period may not seem like a health crisis, it can carry health risks.
If it's linked to hormonal changes, it may affect your bone density, raising your risk for fractures and osteoporosis. It can also make it harder to get pregnant if you're trying.

In most cases, amenorrhea and its underlying causes are treatable. Ask your doctor for more information about your condition, treatment options, and long-term outlook. Please remember if you have no cycle the pill is not the solution and is more than likely pushing the issue further down the line, rather than actually treating things then and there.

If you are coming from an eating disorder background, please know that there is support out there. Please talk to your medical professional or mental health professional.

It is possible to have the life that you want after HA, so please keep the faith and nourish your body.

Chapter 5 - PCOS

What is PCOS?

Polycystic ovary syndrome (PCOS) is the most common hormonal disorder in women. It affects approximately 10% of women of reproductive age worldwide. It is a condition that affects a woman's hormone levels.

PCOS is a combination of things and cannot be solely put down to one only thing. Instead, it needs to be viewed as a set of symptoms. The main symptom is impaired ovulation, leading to androgen excess (Androgens are hormones that contribute to growth and reproduction in both men and women) or a high level of testosterone.

Androgen excess can cause the typical PCOS symptoms of hair growth, hair loss, acne and hirsutism.

A massive note to take before you read any further is that not all women with PCOS are overweight. This is a very common misconception.

PCOS may be diagnosed if **any two** of the following three factors are present:

- A number of cysts have developed around the ovaries (polycystic ovaries)
- A failure in the release of eggs from the ovaries (ovulation)

- Slightly higher than normal levels of LH and Testosterone in your blood

The exact cause is unknown. PCOS is most common in women who are overweight and demonstrate insulin resistance. Insulin resistance appears to be a key factor in PCOS although not all individuals with PCOS possess it. Roughly 70% of those with PCOS are insulin resistant.

Insulin resistance is when the body's tissues don't respond to the normal level of insulin. The body therefore has to produce extra insulin to compensate. This excess insulin can increase the production and activity of LH and Testosterone. The leading result of insulin resistance is excess weight around your midsection.

Insulin is a hormone found in the body that controls glucose (sugar) levels in the blood and allows glucose to be brought into our body's cells to be used as energy.

These can lead to symptoms that vary significantly from woman to woman. These include:

- *Irregular periods* A lack of ovulation prevents the uterine lining from shedding every month. Some women with PCOS get fewer than eight periods a year.
- *Heavy bleeding* the uterine lining builds up for an extended period of time, so the periods you do get can be heavier than normal.
- *Hair growth* More than 70% of women with this condition grow hair on their face and

body — including their back, belly, and chest.
- *Acne* Male hormones can make the skin oilier than usual and cause breakouts on areas like the face, chest, and upper back.
- *Weight gain* Up to 80% of women with PCOS are overweight or obese.
- *Male-pattern baldness* Hair on the scalp gets thinner and falls out.
- *Darkening of the skin* Dark patches of skin can form in body creases like on the neck, the groin, and under the breasts.
- *Headaches* Hormone changes can trigger headaches in some women.

Long term health Risks

In combination with having PCOS and being overweight, PCOS can lead to an increased risk of diabetes, cardiovascular disease, high cholesterol, high blood pressure and fertility problems.

PCOS is one of the most common causes of female infertility. However, many women with PCOS can still conceive. See later on in the chapter for more information on this.

Treating PCOS

Risks can be minimised with a combination of lifestyle changes and adherence to medication.

What can you do?

Weight loss

If you are overweight, even a small amount of weight loss can improve PCOS symptoms.

With PCOS, it is a bit more challenging to lose weight. However, it's not for the reason that you think (lowered Basal Metabolic Rate) that's not to say it does not play a role. It's more to do with appetite regulation, binge eating, and mood issues. More evidence is needed on this before a definitive answer can be made.

It's imperative that you are in the right place to diet. This means that if you have been binge eating, yo-yo dieting etc. you will need to check in with your Doctor, Nutritionist, Dietitian to ensure you are in the right position to diet.

It's not the end if you can't right now. Loss of total body weight can help normalise menstrual cycles, regulate blood sugar, improve self-esteem, reduce depressive symptoms and increase a woman's chances of conceiving a baby.

Consistency is the key to this. It can be incredibly stressful and challenging but difficult but it is so important. Unfortunately, like life there is no quick fix.

Here are some tips that may help:

Eat regular meals

It will help to keep your insulin levels stable throughout the day. Eating often can also help to control your appetite. Try to be aware of recognising signs of hunger and fullness. Developing this consciousness can prevent binge eating (loss of control) or overeating (could stop if the person wanted to). Pre-planning meals also plays a major role in this.

Eat a Balanced Diet

A balanced diet includes eating lots of fruit and vegetables, choosing low-fat dairy foods and lean meats and fish. It's also critical to reduce the amount of fatty, sugary and processed foods and drinks you consume.

Starchy Foods

Studies comparing diets for PCOS have found that lower-carbohydrate diets are effective for weight loss and lowering insulin levels. A low glycaemic index (low-GI) diet that gets most carbohydrates from fruits, vegetables, and whole grains helps regulate the menstrual cycle better than a regular weight loss diet.

Limit Added Sugar

It's critical to avoid high sugar foods with PCOS. Eating less sugar results in lower blood glucose levels. Which decreases insulin levels and reduces male hormone levels. Most women with PCOS crave sugary foods, even after eating meals. This is due to increases in insulin. To best manage insulin levels and reduce the amount of sugar in your diet. Ultimately, it's not sugar that someone is craving. It could be an emotion, tiredness, stress that is present. Please check back to the PMS chapter for the Food and Mood Journal.

Dealing with Cravings

Try fruit instead of sugary foods during sugar cravings. Avoiding sugar, where possible, in your diet will result in fewer cravings for sugar over time. Be sure to eat often, such as every 3 to 5 hours. Have sufficient protein with meals and snacks – this will help with feeling full and aiming for whole grain and complex carbs (e.g., 100 percent whole-wheat breads, Barley, Quinoa, Potatoes).

Around times when hunger increases, it is essential to fuel your body and understand that it is not sugar or carbs that you are craving. There is more than likely an emotion present that is fuelling this. So, it is essential to provide yourself with foods you enjoy each day like chocolate, eat 200-300 extra calories (more if needed) if you are feeling hungrier.

Fats

Some fats are essential in your diet. It is crucial to cut down on saturated fat, e.g., processed meats, pastry, chocolate, cake, biscuits and full-fat dairy products.

Choose lean red meat, poultry without the skin, and the fat cut off. Try to have at least 2-3 servings of oily fish per week, e.g., mackerel, sardines, salmon, pilchards. Omega 3 Fatty Acids will help massively.

One substitute could be unsaturated fats or oils sparingly in cooking – these are more "heart-healthy", e.g. rapeseed or olive oil.

The intake of Alpha Linoleic Acid (Flaxseed, Tofu and Soybeans) positively affects the menstrual regularity of women with PCOS.

Stress & Sleep

Stress can worsen your PCOS symptoms. The stress hormones make your body pump out more testosterone, which can increase insulin resistance. Managing your stress levels is an integral part of getting to grips with your PCOS. Ensure you get enough sleep. Those with PCOS may be more susceptible to Sleep Apnoea than those without it.

Where you can make sure your pre-bed routine is on point. This means limiting screen time, limiting caffeine intake (before 1 pm), and if you are an overthinker, having a pad or a journal beside your bed to write those thoughts onto a page may help.

Suppose you aren't getting enough sleep (ideally 7-9 hours of quality sleep). In that case, your hunger hormones (Ghrelin mainly) will increase, and your fullness hormone activity will decrease. You are creating a scenario where you are more likely to reach for more sugary foods and the vicious cycle will continue.

Exercise

Exercise is also a great way of reducing your stress levels and simultaneously targeting your weight. There are many benefits to be gained from being physically active, including improving insulin resistance. A mixture of Resistance training or HIIT may improve Insulin sensitivity and burn glucose. HIIT may not be the solution if you are stressed and tired all of the time.

Contraception

Hormonal contraception such as the pill, the Mirena IUD, and the depo injection (hereafter also referred to as 'the pill') was not designed to 'regulate your cycle and it can never do this for the simple reason that a menstrual cycle is far more than a bleed.

The bleed is only one tiny part of the menstrual cycle. The reason why you aren't getting a period on your own, or why it's so irregular is because your body is struggling to ovulate. Switching off ovulation altogether via the pill isn't the answer, getting to the root cause of your PCOS is. Additionally, the pill can make things worse for you in the long run.

Unbeknownst to most women, the pill can actually cause insulin resistance – a huge contributory factor in worsening PCOS symptoms. Studies have shown that the pill causes a 30-40% reduction in insulin sensitivity and also stops exercise from improving insulin sensitivity.

One of the major signs of PCOS is irregular periods or completely absent periods, caused by failure to ovulate.

Conventional treatment of PCOS is an oral contraceptive pill, which suppresses the body's ability to ovulate. So absolutely not fixing the problem, it's more than likely sticking a band aid over a broken arm.

Often, GPs will prescribe the pill and tell you to come back when you want to have a baby. Not helpful!

All this is doing is masking the problem and kicking the can down the road to deal with at a later date. When a woman then comes off the pill to have a baby, her stress is through the roof as there is no sign of her period.

This just creates unnecessary pressure when ovulation could have been re-established much earlier on with the help of nutrition and lifestyle changes.

The pill will reduce androgen levels which is why it's great for acne, but it only works for as long as you take it. Often when people come off the pill, they have worse acne and hair growth than before.

So, as you can see, all the pill is doing is brushing the problem under the rug! Instead, I recommend getting to the bottom of what's driving your PCOS and managing it with improvements in nutrition and lifestyle rather than taking the pill.

If you are concerned with this, please talk to a dietician or a doctor.

Fertility & PCOS

PCOS interrupts the normal menstrual cycle and makes it harder to get pregnant. Between 70% and 80% of women with PCOS have fertility problems. This does not make it impossible; it may just mean being more patient and looking at options with your doctor.

Having PCOS doesn't mean you can't get pregnant. It just might be a bit trickier and you may need extra help. You can do plenty at home and with medical treatment to keep PCOS symptoms at bay and raise your chances for a healthy pregnancy.

<u>First steps</u>

- Check-in with Doc to see where hormone levels are at (e.g., thyroid, testosterone)
- Manage your stress levels
- Start eating a decent nutritious diet and exercise plan. Get into the habit of choosing healthier food choices and being more active.
- Use an ovulation calendar or app to track when you have your period. This helps you better guess about which days of the month you are more likely to get pregnant.
- Check your blood sugar levels.

How much does weight play a role?

Being overweight has been linked to PCOS, but many women who have this condition are not overweight. Still, if you are carrying extra weight, you may improve your fertility and reduce other

PCOS symptoms by losing just 5 percent of your weight.

Exercise daily by going for a walk and getting in your steps and even try to get a decent weights program from a qualified coach. Lifting weights will help with bone health and overall health.

Eat for health

A varied diet is key and any woman who is trying to get pregnant needs to have the right levels of nutrients. Certain vitamins and minerals are important for a healthy pregnancy and a growing baby. Ask your doctor about the best supplements for you. Supplements that may help fertility include:

- Folic acid (vitamin B9)
- Vitamin B6
- Vitamin B12
- Vitamin C
- Vitamin D
- Vitamin E
- Coenzyme Q10
- Selenium

Balance blood sugar levels

Your doctor will test your blood sugar levels if you're having trouble getting pregnant. PCOS sometimes leads to high blood sugar levels or type 2 diabetes. This may cause fertility problems.

This happens because PCOS may change how your body uses insulin. PCOS makes your body less sensitive to insulin — making it harder for it to do its job.

Balancing your blood sugar levels may help you get pregnant. Eat a healthy diet with more fibre, protein, and healthy fats. Getting plenty of daily exercise and strength training can also help your body use insulin better.

In some cases, your doctor might recommend medications to help balance your blood sugar levels. A common type 2 diabetes drug called Metformin (or Glucophage) makes your body use insulin better to help lower high blood sugar. Which in turn can also help you get pregnant.

Depending on your blood sugar levels you might need to take metformin in low doses and only temporarily. For best results, eat a healthy diet and exercise regularly along with taking any prescribed medications to help manage your PCOS and if you are looking to start a family down the line, please try to manage your symptoms now rather than pushing it down the line.

Medications

If you have PCOS your body might make more testosterone and estrogen. Too much (or too little) of these hormones can make it tricky to get pregnant. Your doctor might recommend prescription medications to help balance your hormones. (You will need to check with your doctor before going on these)

Medications to help you get pregnant with PCOS include:

- Metformin to balance insulin levels
- Clomiphene citrate (or Clomid) to help balance estrogen levels
- Birth control pills to balance estrogen and testosterone levels (before beginning fertility treatment)
- Fertility medications to jump-start the ovaries to send out more eggs

There is Fertility help out there

You may need in vitro fertilization (IVF) treatment to help you get pregnant with PCOS. Your fertility doctor will give you a check-up that may include more blood tests, ultrasounds scans, and a physical exam.

IVF is a process that can take months or even years whether you have PCOS or not. However, medical research shows that women with PCOS have a high success rate of getting pregnant with IVF treatment.

For all women, the first step in IVF treatment is to eat a balanced diet and get plenty of exercise to reach a healthy weight. Women with PCOS who are a healthy weight are twice as likely to get pregnant with IVF than women with PCOS who are obese.

PCOS symptoms and complications

PCOS may make it harder to get pregnant because it can impact your menstruation cycle (your monthly period). Symptoms include:

- Too few menstrual periods
- Having your period for longer than usual

- Not getting your period
- Very heavy periods
- Higher levels of male hormones like testosterone
- Acne breakouts
- Getting facial hair and extra hair in other places
- Small cysts or bundles of fluid in the ovaries
- Fewer eggs released from the ovaries

No one knows why some women get PCOS. Nothing you did — or didn't do— caused you to have this condition. But getting an early diagnosis and treatment along with making other lifestyle changes may help you get pregnant and prevent health complications from PCOS.

You can get pregnant with PCOS. You will likely need to have moderate weight, balance your blood sugar levels, and treat other PCOS symptoms with healthy lifestyle changes and medications.

In some cases, fertility medications alone will help you get pregnant. If that doesn't work, you may need IVF treatment.

But regardless of what treatment you explore, don't lose hope. Speak to your doctor or dietitian about this.

Main types of PCOS

There are four main types of PCOS. It is so important to understand the type that you or your client may have. Otherwise, it is like throwing paint at a wall and hoping something sticks.

The four main types are Insulin-Resistant PCOS, Post Pill PCOS, Inflammatory PCOS, and Adrenal PCOS.

Let's start with the most common form, Insulin Resistant PCOS.

Insulin resistant PCOS

The most common type of PCOS, affecting around 70% of those with PCOS. Insulin resistance is higher insulin levels than normal in the body - also known as hyperinsulinemia. This happens when our cells become a bit "numb" to the effects of insulin, which causes the pancreas to pump out more and more insulin until the cells get the message.

In this type of PCOS, you may be struggling with your weight, holding weight around the stomach/abdomen, having more cravings, and symptoms like fatigue or brain fog. It's high insulin levels that drive up androgen levels, which cause issues like excess hair, male pattern hair loss, and acne.

Testing for Insulin Resistance

- Often doctors will test HbA1c or glucose levels, which gives us some information about your blood sugar levels but doesn't give us the complete picture. To rule out insulin resistance, you NEED to have your fasting insulin tested. A healthy "fasting insulin" should be less than 10 mIU/L (60

pmol/L). One and two hours after a sugar challenge, a healthy insulin reading should be less than 60 mIU/L (410 pmol/L). High insulin means you have insulin resistance.
- It is highly recommended that you have your waist measured. Insulin resistance PCOS can cause apple-shaped obesity. What this basically means is that the larger your waist circumference, the more likely you are to have insulin resistance. As a woman, your risk starts when your waist circumference is greater than 32 inches (80 cm). Please note that you do not need to be overweight to have insulin resistance.

To help treat insulin resistant PCOS, the key is down to improving your insulin sensitivity. You can work on this through:

1. *Regular exercise and movement throughout the day* which helps your body to burn sugar, build muscle and improve your sensitivity to insulin. The best form of training would involve some sort of weights training and some HIIT (High-Intensity Interval Training) if the body is able to recover from this. Aiming for three times per week is a safe place to start. Exercise improves insulin sensitivity in the muscles by increasing the number of mitochondria, which are the powerhouses of the cell and turn food into energy. Building healthy muscle also requires sufficient dietary protein.
2. *Reducing high sugar foods* (where possible) and having a lower carbohydrate diet that is

also rich in protein and fat to balance blood sugar levels.
3. *Prioritising sleep and reducing stress* can also help to manage blood sugar and insulin levels. Circadian rhythm or body clock has a profound effect on glucose metabolism and whole-body insulin sensitivity, and dysregulation of the circadian rhythm is a contributing cause of insulin resistance.

   The best way to support circadian rhythm is to maintain regular patterns of eating and light exposure (daylight exposure early in the mornings has massive benefits). Watch out for those pesky lights on your phone. Blue light blocking glasses are cheap and an effective way of helping you to protect your sleep alongside keeping digital devices outside of the bedroom.

   Without regular sleep, this can have a massive impact on your hunger signal. It can up-regulate your hunger hormone and down-regulate your fullness hormones. This will make the brain look for the quickest hit of energy and in most cases, carbs and sugary foods are the foods that most go for. There is absolutely nothing wrong with these foods but it is important to have everything in moderation.

4. The best supplements for insulin resistance are Magnesium, Lipoic acid, Inositol, and Berberine can also be extremely helpful. I strongly advise working with a Nutritionist or

Naturopath to find out what is best for you at what dosage, as this will vary from person to person and is key to getting results.

One massive caveat before reading on is the Pill is not a treatment for this type of PCOS (or any type) because it impairs insulin sensitivity. Improvements in this type of PCOS will be slow and gradual and can take up to 6 - 9 months to see any noticeable improvements.

Post-pill PCOS

Post-pill PCOS occurs in some women after they stop taking the oral contraceptive pill. This is due to hormonal birth control suppressing ovulation. For most women this is a temporary effect and ovulation will hopefully resume fairly promptly after the pill is stopped.

But for some women, ovulation suppression can persist for months or even years (please seek medical advice if this is the case).

It is the second most common type of PCOS and more research is needed in this area to get the bigger picture.

Treatment ideas:

If your LH is elevated, the best herbal treatment is Peony & liquorice combination. If your prolactin is high-normal, the best herbal treatment is Vitex (also called chaste tree or chaste berry). Do not use Vitex if your LH is elevated. If you are on medication for mental health, please do not take Vitex.

Both Peony and Vitex work on your pituitary-ovarian axis, and they are powerful herbs. I recommend you do not use them too soon or for too long.

Do not take them if you are a teenager, or have just come off the Pill. Give yourself at least 3-4 months off the Pill.

Do not use Peony or Vitex for more than 10 months in a row. They should not need to be used that way. If they are the right herbs, they will work fairly quickly (within 3-4 months). And then, your periods should stay regular after you stop the herbs. Do not take liquorice if you have high blood pressure. Please seek professional advice.

In this type, symptoms like acne, irregular periods and excess hair growth were not present prior to starting the pill at all then you may have Post Pill PCOS.

Oral contraceptives such as Ginet, Yasmin and Yaz are often involved in this type of PCOS due to synthetic progestins used. After coming off the pill, your ovaries basically throw a party. A natural surge in androgens can cause typical PCOS symptoms; however, there is no insulin resistance in this type.

Keep in mind that this type can take time to heal on its own, but can be addressed more quickly with the right nutrition, lifestyle changes and supplementation or herbal medicine support. It can take up to 3-6 months for this to sync back up together.

Sleep and stress management are huge factors with Post Pill PCOS. It is important to get a good quality sleep and reduce stress levels to support overall hormonal balance.

Adrenal PCOS

This type of PCOS is due to abnormal stress response and affects around 10% of those diagnosed. Typically, DHEA-S (another type of androgen from the adrenal glands) will be elevated alone, and high levels of testosterone and androstenedione are not seen. Unfortunately, this type of androgen isn't often tested unless you go through an endocrinologist or other specialist.

Adrenal PCOS is not driven by insulin resistance or inflammation. Instead, it's an epigenetic upregulation of adrenal androgens. Some research has shown that a natural anti-androgen supplement e.g., Zinc or DIM may work alongside treating the underlying driver of your PCOS.

How will you know if this is you?

If you have ruled out insulin-resistance, and testing shows only your DHEAS is elevated and not your other androgens, then you are most likely dealing with adrenal PCOS.

<u>To help treat adrenal PCOS:</u>

- Manage stress. Reducing stress levels through activities like Yoga, meditation, mindfulness, and journaling will help support your nervous system and hormones. Managing stress levels is essential for overall hormone health.

- Get enough sleep each night. Make sure you're waking up rested and getting 7-9 hours of sleep where possible. My advice is to keep technology out of the bedroom.
- Avoid high-intensity exercise. Limit excessive and high-intensity training as this can further put stress on your adrenals. This will be very person dependent as some people may be able to recover quicker than others.
- Watch intake of caffeine.
- Speak to a practitioner about herbs and supplements. Treatments include magnesium, Zinc, liquorice, adaptogen herbs, and vitamin B5, the "anti-stress factor."
- Give apoptogenic herbs a go, such as Ashwagandha which helps the body 'adapt' to and better respond to stress. These do not get to the root cause of the stress but can help to calm the Central Nervous System (CNS). Please note that Ashwagandha does not solve stress completely. You are better off looking at your lifestyle.

Inflammatory PCOS

In inflammatory PCOS, this is where chronic inflammation causes the ovaries to produce excess testosterone, resulting in physical symptoms and issues with ovulation. Signs of inflammation in this type of PCOS include headaches, joint pain, unexplained fatigue, skin issues like eczema and bowel issues like IBS.

Typically, you will see raised inflammatory markers

on a blood test, such as a high CRP (C reactive protein) above 5. Other tests such as fasting glucose and insulin are in the normal range, but can sometimes be affected as inflammation can affect these numbers.

The key treatment for inflammatory PCOS is to identify and correct the underlying source of inflammation.

To help treat inflammatory PCOS:

- Address gut health. Remove food triggers. Some foods can cause discomfort more than others for some. Some of the main ones can be gluten or dairy. Unless you are lactose intolerant you do not need to eliminate dairy from your diet; it is normally danger in the dose. Addressing potential food sensitivities and the removal of inflammatory foods is a vital step to help address inflammation. It can sometimes be quite difficult to figure out what foods might be driving your inflammation, so it's best to work with a nutritionist or dietitian on this who can help you.
- Look after your gut with Zinc, collagen, l-glutamine and probiotic-rich foods. Probiotic supplements are another treatment for inflammatory PCOS. They help to reduce inflammation and improve gut health. If you have IBS consider the use of the probiotic strain Lactobacillus plantarum 299v. Please seek medical advice or advice with a Dietitian before reaching for a probiotic.

- Supplement with magnesium or melatonin to support sleep and help to calm your nervous system. Other supplements like Zinc and N-acetyl cysteine work particularly well for inflammatory PCOS.
- Natural anti-inflammatories such as turmeric, omega 3 fatty acids, and antioxidants like NAC can help support this type of PCOS. Always speak to a practitioner first to see if these are right for you and what dosages to take for them to be effective.

There is some overlap between these four types. For example, inflammation is a major driver in both the insulin-resistant and inflammatory type of PCOS.

Could it be something else?

PCOS can often be misdiagnosed for something else called Hypothalamic Amenorrhoea (please see the previous chapter for more information). In Hypothalamic Amenorrhoea (HA), your period can stop due to under-eating and/or overexercising, and similarly to PCOS can present itself with mild acne, excess hair growth and a polycystic ovary appearance on an ultrasound. This misdiagnosis is problematic as the treatment of the two conditions are very different.

The main difference between PCOS vs Hypothalamic Amenorrhoea is what is known as the LH: FSH ratio. In PCOS, luteinising hormone (LH) can be 2-3 times higher than follicle stimulating hormone (FSH) when they should be at about a 1:1 ratio. However, in hypothalamic amenorrhoea, the opposite is true, and LH can be much lower than

FSH.

It is so important to know what type of PCOS you have so that you can manage it correctly.

Getting a diagnosis of PCOS

PCOS can be a complex condition to identify because there are numerous symptoms, and you don't have to have all of them to be diagnosed with PCOS. Very few women have the same set of symptoms, and the symptoms can change at different stages of your life.

The symptoms differ widely between women, but the three main areas they affect are:

- fertility and reproductive health
- metabolic health
- psychological health

Although there is no cure for PCOS, the good news is that PCOS is treatable. We know that your lifestyle (what we eat and how active we are) can worsen or improve PCOS symptoms. With support from your doctor and other healthcare givers, there are many ways to manage your lifestyle and improve PCOS aspects.

Criteria for a diagnosis for PCOS

Criteria for a diagnosis of PCOS
A diagnosis of PCOS can be made when at least two of the following three criteria are met:

1. *Irregular periods or no periods*

2. *Higher levels of androgens are present in the blood (hyperandrogenism), shown by:*

- A blood test
- Excess facial or body hair growth
- Hair loss on the scalp
- Acne.

3. *Polycystic ovaries cannot be diagnosed or ruled out by ultrasound*

PCOS cannot be diagnosed by ultrasound because polycystic ovaries are not cysts. They're follicles or eggs, which are normal for the ovary.

It's normal for all women to sometimes have a higher number of follicles. It's normal for young women to always have a higher number of follicles because young women have more eggs.

That's why PCOS cannot be diagnosed by ultrasound.

At the same time, PCOS cannot be ruled out by ultrasound because it's possible to have normal-appearing ovaries on ultrasound and still have the hormonal condition PCOS.

In women younger than 20 years, ultrasounds are not recommended. This means that irregular periods and hyperandrogenism need to be present for PCOS diagnosis to be made.
A number of other conditions that could cause

similar symptoms of irregular periods or no periods need to be checked by your doctor and ruled out before a correct diagnosis of PCOS can be confirmed.

4. *Watch out for temporary PCOS*

Polycystic ovaries, irregular cycles, high androgens (male hormones), and even mild insulin resistance are all normal and healthy during puberty. That's why now experts recommend that PCOS not be diagnosed until at least three years after the onset of periods. So, if you are a teenager, please wait for at least three years after the onset of your period.

If you are feeling discomfort or pain then it may be something else. So please check with a medical professional on this.

Post-pill PCOS is a temporary state of androgen excess when coming off the pill. It happens for several reasons:

- Coming off an androgen-suppressing contraceptive drug such as drospirenone (Yasmin) can cause a temporary surge in androgens, which can lead to a PCOS diagnosis. Given time, post-pill PCOS usually resolves.
- Hormonal birth control can cause or worsen insulin resistance and is a major contributor to classic insulin-resistant PCOS.
- Hormonal birth control disrupts the healthy signalling of the HPO (hypothalamic-

pituitary-ovarian) axis, making it hard to resume ovulation once stopping the pill.

It is so important that you get the correct diagnosis of your PCOS.

5. *Diagnosis of PCOS*

Right now, there is no definitive test to diagnose PCOS. Your doctor will more than likely start with a discussion of your medical history, including your cycle regularity and any noticeable weight changes. They may recommend an ultrasound. This can neither confirm or deny PCOS.

Your doctor may also recommend:

- A pelvic exam to examine manually reproductive organs, growth or for any abnormalities.
- Blood tests. This can rule out any possible causes of menstrual abnormalities or androgen excess that may mimic PCOS.
- Dutch test. This is the most advanced hormone test. This will need to be done privately so it may be more expensive financially. The DUTCH test stands for Dried Urine Test for Comprehensive Hormones and involves collection of a small amount of urine on filtered paper four times a day. The DUTCH TEST measures hormone metabolites from the dried urine samples. The hormones measured in the test include:
    - Cortisol
    - Cortisone

- Estradiol
- Estrone
- Estriol
- Progesterone
- Testosterone
- DHEA
- Melatonin

While hormone blood tests are a helpful tool, they are not the same as the DUTCH test. Blood and saliva tests don't measure cortisol rhythms and estrogen metabolism and do not track hormone replacement as thoroughly, not being sensitive enough to see the different levels of estrogen, which can be an issue for women when it comes to trying to figure out their estrogen state, and can impact on their overall health.

What makes the DUTCH test better than blood or saliva tests is the comprehensive information that is collected.

The Dutch test can be great for identifying fertility problems, including PCOS. It provides a comprehensive picture of how the adrenal and reproductive hormone imbalances may be contributing to these problems.

Ideally the DUTCH test or sex hormone test is done on days 19, 20, 21, or 22 (or 5-7 days after ovulation is the goal) if the first day of bleeding is considered day 1.

Are there best times to test hormone levels?

If you are struggling with a hormone imbalance, testing your sex hormones can help you understand where your issue is rooted and see what is driving your symptoms.

Hormone levels are like stock prices; they fluctuate throughout the month and this is why so many women get "within range" test results. So, let's start with estrogen.

What day should estrogen levels be checked?

When evaluating female estrogen levels, day 3 is when estradiol, along with follicle stimulating hormone (FSH) and luteinizing hormone (LH) blood tests will be performed. Testing at the beginning of the cycle, along with FSH can help us understand brain-ovarian communication. Measuring FSH and LH is important to assess how the brain is talking to the ovaries.

When Should FSH Levels Be Checked?

For fertility or evaluating ovarian reserve, FSH is tested on day 3 of your cycle. If you cannot have lab testing done, most providers are fine testing between days 2-4. Testing on or around day 3 of your cycle can be helpful in evaluating PCOS diagnosis as well. **Please note**, this test alone will not diagnose PCOS.

FSH and LH can help us understand how the brain

is talking to the ovaries and the hormones can help us know how the ovaries respond to that message.

Why Test Estradiol?

During your reproductive years, estradiol or E2 is the predominant form of estrogen. As women transition into menopause, estrone or E1 becomes the most common circulating estrogen. This is important to understand because depending on the phase of life you are in, your estrogen levels and the type of estrogen will vary. If you are in a phase of life where you should be having periods, you need to check estradiol.

What days to test Estrogen?

Checking estrogen levels around day three (third day of your period) and in some cases, between days 19-22 or roughly 5-7 days after ovulation is recommended. Evaluating your estrogen levels, especially in relation to progesterone during the luteal phase can help you identify if your symptoms like weight gain, irritability, and heavy periods are related to estrogen dominance.

When you simply test on the day you happen to be in the doctor's office getting an exam, your levels may be just fine for that particular day. To get a really good understanding of estrogen levels and how they're affecting your symptoms, you have to test and compare with where they should be based on the timing of your cycle.

When to test Progesterone?

Progesterone levels are highest 5-7 days following ovulation, which is within your luteal phase (the second half of your cycle). This is why testing is recommended on days 19-22 of a 28-day cycle.

Even though women are told that they ovulate like clockwork on day 14 of their cycle, unfortunately, this isn't always the case. In fact, roughly 12% of women have a 28 day cycle.

It's a great idea to track your basal body temperature and evaluate your cervical mucus to get an idea of when and if you are ovulating. When you ovulate, your body temperature rises and your vaginal discharge becomes the consistency of egg whites. If you keep an eye on these changes to your body, there's a pretty good chance you can approximate when you're ovulating.

For a lot of women, this will mean they should test for progesterone between days 19-22 of their cycle. Again, this recommendation could change if you're not ovulating day 14 of your cycle — which is actually pretty common, or if your typical cycle is shorter or longer than 28 days. Track your cycle for a few months before and talk to your doctor so that they can tell you the best day to test progesterone. If you feel confused, talk to the provider ordering your test.

Tracking your cycle through apps like Natural Cycles, Clue, Kindara or keeping a note on a notebook will help you to understand your body.

When to test Testosterone?

Yes, testosterone is a key hormone to test for women.

When testosterone levels are low, we often see low libido, fatigue, and even depression. And when they're high, as we often see in polycystic ovarian syndrome (PCOS), women experience acne, irregular periods, and hair growth on the chin, chest and abdomen. Elevated testosterone can also lead to hair loss on the scalp.

Testosterone levels vary by age — so results have to be interpreted accordingly. You have to test BOTH total and free testosterone and sex hormone-binding globulin (SHBG) to get a clear picture of what exactly is going on.

You can get your testosterone levels measured any time of the month, but this test is best done in the morning because that is when levels are highest.

What do I test if I don't have a period?

If your period has stopped showing up (or never arrived in the first place), this is what is called Amenorrhea.
Primary amenorrhea is when you haven't gotten your period by age 15 or 16.

Secondary amenorrhea is when you have had a period, but now it's gone. (If your regular period is missing for three or more months, or your irregular period is missing for six or more months, this is considered secondary amenorrhea.)

Often, doctors will try to prescribe the birth control pill as a means of "treating" amenorrhea. If they do this is not the solution so, please get a second opinion.

If you begin birth control, you will not be able to test FSH, LH, estradiol or progesterone accurately.

The Endocrine Society guidelines clearly advocate against the use of the pill in women with functional hypothalamic amenorrhea solely to restore a period or even improve bone mass. They also recommend educating patients who are currently using the pill that it may mask these issues.

Lab Test to Consider for a Missing Period

- Pregnancy test
- Progesterone
- Estrogen
- FSH
- LH
- Testosterone
- SHBG
- TSH
- T4
- T3
- B12
- Ferritin
- Folate
- Prolactin

Will you need all of these? Maybe. Maybe not.

This is where an experienced clinician can help. If you find that when you talk to your doctor or medical professional, they are hesitant to test these, remember you are fully entitled to get these tested. If they make you feel uncomfortable, please go elsewhere.

Also — don't let a doctor convince you that a missing period doesn't matter because you're not interested in baby-making at the moment. Amenorrhea is a sign of an underlying issue that needs to be addressed, whether you're trying to conceive or not. The quality of care you receive should not be dependent on whether or not you want to have a baby at this moment.

When is the best time to test other hormone levels?

Your sex hormones aren't the only ones you may need to look at to understand the cause of your hormone symptoms.

When to Test Insulin?

If you're trying to get to the bottom of a PCOS diagnosis, you will need to evaluate insulin. If you have a family history of diabetes or your clinician suspects insulin dysregulation, this is a test they will likely order. Typically, insulin is tested while fasting along with blood glucose. Because of this, the test is commonly done first thing in the morning.

A healthy "fasting insulin" should be less than 10 mIU/L (60 pmol/L). One and two hours after a sugar challenge, a healthy insulin reading should be less than 60 mIU/L (410 pmol/L). High insulin means you have insulin resistance.

Your doctor will help determine the right tests for you.

When to Test Cortisol?

We can't always get a full picture of what's going on with your hormones without looking at the adrenals, which produce the stress hormone cortisol. Cortisol is involved in your stress response, hair loss, blood sugar regulation, and more. In times of stress, the body will shift into preferentially making cortisol over progesterone.

Cortisol blood tests are best performed in the morning, along with Adrenocorticotropic hormone (ACTH), because this is when levels are highest. ACTH is produced in the pituitary gland and helps your adrenals to function. For a more comprehensive picture of adrenal function, salivary or urinary cortisol is best. Cortisol can be tested at any time of the month.

If you know you are feeling stressed you probably don't need a test to tell you that your cortisol is high. It could be an idea to look at the root cause of your stress, for example work, family or finances.

When to Test DHEA?

Dehydroepiandrosterone (DHEA) is a crucial anti-ageing hormone the body can convert into estrogen or testosterone. It is an essential marker of adrenal function and is a hormone that declines with age. DHEA can be tested at any time of the month and is typically done alongside a cortisol test.

When to Test Thyroid?

We can't discuss testing for hormone imbalances without looking at the thyroid (please check the Thyroid chapter for more information). Thyroid testing is best down first thing in the morning and can be at any point in your cycle. It's important to stop any supplements with biotin at least 72 hours in advance as it can skew results. At a minimum, I would suggest looking at:

- Thyroid-stimulating hormone (TSH): a brain hormone which signals your thyroid to produce T4 (& a little bit of T3). A lot of doctors will test TSH only, which doesn't give the full picture of thyroid function.
- Free Thyroxine (T4) and Free Triiodothyronine (T3)
- Thyroid binding globulin (TBG): a protein which transports thyroid hormone in the bloodstream. When thyroid hormone is bound it is measured via blood test as Total T4 & Total T3. Your cells use Free T4 & Free T3. This is why we measure both of these markers in addition to TSH. Your T4 is inactive and T3 is active. T3 is involved in your mood, menses, metabolism, and gut motility.
- Thyroid peroxidase (TPO) and Thyroglobulin (TgAb) antibodies: the most common antibodies to see with Hashimoto's

hypothyroidism and the most common cause of hypothyroidism. Often, antibodies will present prior to symptoms of thyroid dysfunction.
- Thyroid Receptor Antibodies: seen in cases of hyperthyroidism or Graves' disease. This condition is less common and so this test is only ordered when clinical suspicion is high.
- Reverse T3: considered inactive thyroid hormone that can be elevated in times of stress, both physical and emotional. The goal here is to measure at minimum TSH, Free T4, and T3 so you get a picture of what the brain says, how the thyroid responds, and the body's ability to activate the thyroid hormone you actually use.

It's extremely important to work with a doctor to interpret your thyroid test results. Abnormal thyroid labs don't necessarily indicate a thyroid problem.

Sometimes, other things going on in your body can look like thyroid dysfunction. If there's a deeper issue at play, simply evaluating your thyroid and stopping there could lead to an insufficient diagnosis.

It's also important to note that the pill's role in elevating Thyroid binding globulin (TBG), Sex Hormone Binding Globulin (SHBG), and Cortisol Binding Globulin (CBG) is well recognized. In fact, it is how researchers can verify who is and isn't actually taking the pill in clinical trials.

When TBG goes up, total thyroid hormone levels go up, and free thyroid levels can go down.

Now, if you thought total thyroid hormone was what the body utilized & that is all you measured, then you might think, "thyroid function is improved on birth control." However, FREE thyroid hormone is what you use, and not bound thyroid hormone (TOTAL). ☐ This is why it is encouraged to test thyroid hormones before someone starts the pill and working alongside your medical professional you continue to monitor symptoms.

Hidden Drivers of PCOS

Many things can impair ovulation and promote excess androgens and these include:

- Thyroid Disease - this is mainly due to hypothyroidism impending ovulation and it can also worsen insulin resistance
- Vitamin D deficiency - ovaries need Vitamin D
- Zinc deficiency - ovaries need Zinc
- Iodine deficiency - ovaries need iodine (please check with your doctor before taking iodine if you have issues with your thyroid)
- Elevated prolactin - this can increase Dehydroepiandrosterone (DHEA) and this is a crucial anti-aging hormone that the body can convert into estrogen or testosterone
- Carbs intake is low - Contrary to a lot of information we have grown up with, Carbs are essential for hormone health and for ovulation. If you're undereating, then you have more than likely slipped into HA (Hypothalamic Amenorrhea).

Supplements to aid PCOS

It is important to note that the point of any supplement is to supplement a diet and lifestyle not the other way around. Please double check with your doctor regarding any of the supplements suggested below.

Myo Inositol

The evidence base around Inositol (and the safety of its use) is too compelling to ignore anymore. These are the possible beneficial effects:

- Reduction of insulin resistance
- Reduction of blood androgen levels
- Improving cardiovascular risk
- Regularisation of the menstrual cycle with spontaneous ovulation.

A recent study showed D-chiro-supplementation alone may not be beneficial because while Myo-inositol may be converted to D-chiro, D-chiro-inositol cannot raise levels of Myo-inositol. In this study the current position supports combined therapy of Myo-inositol and D-chiro-inositol administered in the physiological ratio of 40:1, which ensures better clinical results. Thus, combination therapy has the advantage of providing small physiological levels. More research is needed on this.

I have seen amazing results with clients with supplementation of 2-4g per day of Myo-inositol. Take it daily for 6 months alongside eating well and exercising. Ideally 2x2g servings a day.

Berberine

Berberine has done well in clinical trials outperforming metformin in two very large studies. Generally, this can be a very good treatment for those suffering from acne and has the added benefit of reducing anxiety. It helps to improve insulin sensitivity, possibly by its benefit on gut bacteria. Berberine also promotes ovulation and helps to prevent the ovaries from taking too much testosterone.

Do not take Berberine if you are pregnant or breastfeeding. Please consult with your doctor if you are combining with prescription medications such as antidepressants, beta-blockers, antibiotics or immunosuppressants because it can alter the level of these medications.

Do not take Berberine for more than 8 weeks as it could alter the composition of your gut bacteria. Please seek medical advice before taking this.

The recommended dose is X3 500mg per day.

For berberine, however, recent studies have been shown only with the addition of metformin. At this juncture, current evidence for an isolated therapy would favour inositol over berberine.

Acetyl-l-carnitine

In one study, the data showed a significant improvement in insulin sensitivity and decreases in serum LDL levels, serum HDL levels and BMI after three months of treatment. More regular menstrual cycles and decreased hirsutism were also observed.

It appears that treatment with L-carnitine might decrease the risk of cardiovascular events by normalizing metabolic profiles and BMI.

2g per day is the recommended intake.

Magnesium

Magnesium can help to improve insulin sensitivity. Usually, a recommendation of 100-300mg per day directly after food. Magnesium supplementation is used generally in neurologic disorders, including depression-related diseases such as PCOS, as well hypertension, cardiovascular diseases, and diabetes. More research is needed for this as some data has shown benefits.

Magnesium deficiency is a significant contributor to insulin resistance. Fortunately, taking magnesium has been found to improve insulin resistance. Magnesium has many benefits, including regulating the HPA (Hypothalamus-pituitary and adrenal) axis, improving sleep, supporting progesterone, curbing sugar cravings, and reducing inflammation.

Vitamin D

There have been many studies suggesting that a lack of vitamin D leads to insulin resistance. Supplementing with vitamin D may help to prevent this, however, more research is needed before this can be confirmed. In general, you would be looking at 2000iu a day.

Vitamin B

Vitamin B12 helps keep the body's nerves and blood cells healthy and helps make DNA. Many women with PCOS are prescribed Metformin. Unfortunately, Metformin can reduce the absorption of vitamin B12 and lead to a B12 deficiency and, subsequently, anaemia. Women taking Metformin should get their B12 levels checked regularly and consider taking a supplement.

Please do not take all of these together; it will depend on the type of PCOS that you have. Please see earlier in the chapter to review which type you may have.

What about the Pill and PCOS?

The Pill deserves a whole chapter by itself and that is why it is important that you read the chapter on the pill. The pill is one of those things that a lot of women need to understand that it is their decision whether they take it or not. It's your body and no one can make you take it if you don't wish to.

Some doctors may prescribe the pill to manage symptoms like heavy, painful periods, hormonal imbalance, acne (won't solve it long term), irregular periods, excess hair growth and lack of ovulation. In order to make the decision you need to have all of the information available to you.

So, the main types of birth control that doctors to suggest to use to help manage PCOS are:

- Oral Contraceptives
- Combination Pill
- Progestin-only Pill
- Skin Patch
- Vaginal Ring

Now let's look into why each one is suggested and how each one works (for more detail please head over to the Chapter on the Pill).

Oral contraceptives

Oral contraceptives are the most common and effective option used to manage PCOS symptoms. There are two types of oral contraceptives: combination pills and progestin-only pills.

Both types of birth control are effective for treating some of the following PCOS symptoms:

- have regular periods
- have lighter periods
- reduce cramping
- have clearer skin
- lower your risks for endometrial cancer, ovarian cancer, and ovarian cysts
- reduce extra hair growth

Most women who have PCOS don't experience side effects when taking the pill, but different types of birth control affect everyone differently. You may experience one or more of the following:

- mood changes
- possible weight gain or loss

- nausea
- headaches
- sore breasts
- some spotting

Combination pill

Combination pills contain estrogen and progestin which are two synthetic (artificial) hormones. The amount of hormone present varies from brand to brand. Your doctor will help determine the right dosage for you.

Progestin-only pill

Progestin-only pills, known as mini pills, are an effective alternative for women who have PCOS and are unable to take combination birth control pills. PCOS causes you to have low levels of the hormone progesterone. They can aid in you having more regular periods and lower your risk of endometrial cancer.

Skin patch

The contraceptive patch is a thin plastic patch that contains estrogen and progestin. You wear the patch for 21 days, remove it for seven days to allow for a menstrual period, then replace it with a new patch. Like the pill, the patch can help you:

- regulate your periods
- reduce bloating and cramps
- reduce acne
- reduce excess hair growth

- lower your cancer risk

Vaginal ring

The contraceptive ring (NuvaRing) is a soft, flexible plastic ring that you insert into your vagina. You wear the ring for 21 days, remove it for seven days to allow for a period, and then replace it with a new one for the next month. Like the pill and the patch, the vaginal ring can help you:

- regulate your periods
- reduce bloating and cramps
- reduce acne
- reduce excess body hair
- lower your cancer risk

Will any form of hormonal birth control work?

Combination birth control — whether in the form of a pill, ring, or patch — is the most popular and recommended form of treatment for PCOS. If you're unable to take the combination pill or use other combination methods, your doctor may recommend the progestin-only pill. There are also other alternatives, including:

- *Progesterone therapy:* You can take progesterone for 10 to 14 days every one to two months. This treatment doesn't prevent pregnancy or improve androgen levels, but it can help manage your symptoms.
- *Progestin-containing intrauterine device (IUD)*: IUDs that contain progestin can help

ease the symptoms of PCOS in the same way combination or progestin-only pills do.
- *Metformin*: This medication is for type 2 diabetes which lowers insulin and androgen levels and improves insulin resistance. Insulin resistance commonly occurs with PCOS, and metformin might be used to treat this.

Choosing the best option for you

If you have PCOS, talk to your doctor about what treatment option would be best for you. When you and your doctor work through your options, remember to consider:

- Ease of use
- Side effects
- Cost

Once you know what you are dealing with and you know the driver then a remedy can be put into place and symptoms can improve quickly. It could be a better option to manage the symptoms rather than using a pill. Your doctor will hopefully provide you with all of the information but if you are unhappy with what has been prescribed you have the right to seek a second opinion and to ask lots of questions.

Treatments of Facial Hair, Acne and Female Pattern Hair Loss

Facial Hair, Acne and Female Pattern Hair Loss are all common symptoms of PCOS but they can also occur for other reasons. The treatments suggested below are for those with or without PCOS.

Why does PCOS cause hair loss?

The female body produces male hormones, also called androgens. This includes testosterone. Androgens play a role in triggering puberty and stimulating hair growth in the underarms and pubic areas. They have other important functions as well.

PCOS causes extra androgen production, resulting in virilization. This refers to the development of more masculine features, including excess hair in places where it doesn't usually grow, such as the:

- Face
- Neck
- Chest
- Abdomen

These extra androgens can also cause the hair on your head to start thinning, especially near the front of your scalp. This is known as androgenic alopecia or female pattern hair loss.

Will it grow back?

Any hair that you lose due to PCOS won't grow back on its own. But, with treatment, you may be able to stimulate the growth of new hair. Plus, there are several things you can do to mask PCOS-related hair loss.

Can medical treatments help?

PCOS hair loss is caused by a hormonal imbalance, so hormone regulation is an important part of treatment. This can be done with a variety of medications which a medical professional can help guide you on.

Keep in mind that you may need to play around with a few different medications before you find one that works for you. And most people have the best results with a combination of medication.

Here's a look at some common treatment options for PCOS-related hair loss.

<u>Oral contraceptive pills</u>

Birth control pills can lower androgen levels, which may help to reduce excess hair growth and slow down hair loss. It also helps with other PCOS symptoms, such as irregular periods and acne. An anti-androgen drug is often prescribed in combination with oral contraceptives for PCOS-related hair loss.

Some conventional anti-androgen treatments include the drugs cyproterone (Androcur) and Spironolactone (Aldactone).

Other natural anti-androgen treatments include:

- Zinc
- DIM (diindolylmethane)
- Micronized or natural progesterone

- Vitex or Agnus Castus

Please note that you do not use all of these supplements. Start with the core treatments mentioned earlier in the chapter.

Spironolactone (Aldactone)

Spironolactone is an oral medication that's known as an aldosterone receptor antagonist. It can be effective for treating androgenetic alopecia. Please talk to your medical professional about spironolactone.

It blocks the effects of androgen on the skin and is usually prescribed together with an oral contraceptive.

Minoxidil (Rogaine)

Minoxidil is the only FDA-approved drug for treating female pattern baldness. It's a topical treatment that you apply to your scalp daily. It promotes hair growth and can even give it a thicker appearance. Please talk to your medical professional about Minoxidil (Rogaine).

While there's some evidence that these drugs can help with female pattern hair loss, many experts don't consider them a good option based on mixed results in other studies and known side effects in women.

What about home remedies?

If you're looking to go the more natural route, some home remedies may help to reduce androgen levels, lessening their effect on your hair.

Zinc

Taking a zinc supplement may help with PCOS-related hair loss, according to a 2016 study. The study looked at the effects of zinc supplementation on PCOS and found that using 50 mg of elemental zinc daily for 8 weeks had a beneficial impact on hair loss. It was also found to help hirsutism.

Weight loss

There's significant evidence that losing weight can lower androgen levels and reduce the effects of excess androgens in women with PCOS. This can lead to less hair loss, as well as a reduction in other PCOS symptoms.

Losing just 5 to 10 percent of your body weight can significantly reduce PCOS symptoms. Not everyone has to lose weight, and this is a personal preference if you wish to do so. Everyone has the right to look and feel like they want. If someone has done extreme dieting for a lot of their life then weight loss may not be the solution. You must be in the right headspace.

Biotin

Biotin is a popular supplement that's often used for

hair health and growth. There's not much evidence that it helps specifically with PCOS-related hair loss, but it may be worth a try. More research is needed on this.

Acne

In addition to affecting a woman's fertility, PCOS can cause several hormone-induced side effects, including acne.

Although conversations about PCOS often focus on the noncancerous growths it causes, hormonal imbalance is at the heart of the condition.

Your body depends on signals from your pituitary gland to produce the right amounts of estrogen, progesterone, and testosterone. PCOS disrupts these signals. So, it's crucial to be aware of the type of PCOS you have to manage it. Please check the beginning of the chapter to see what type you have.

Without the right signals from the pituitary gland, your estrogen and progesterone levels drop, and your testosterone levels increase.

This can prevent ovulation and lead to symptoms like:

- Irregular menstruation.
- Acne.
- Hair growth on your face, chest, or back (hirsutism).
- Weight gain or difficulty losing weight.

- Patches of dark skin on the back of your neck or other areas.

<u>What else causes acne?</u>

PCOS is just one of many risk factors for acne.

In general, acne is caused by:

- Excess oil production.
- Dead skin cells trapped deep in your pores.
- Bacteria.
- Excess hormone activity.

Acne may also result from:

- Stress.
- Hormonal changes, such as during pregnancy.
- Certain medications, such as corticosteroids (please talk to a medical professional if you are taking medications and you feel they are causing acne).

Certain behaviours can also increase your risk for acne, which include:

- Not washing your face regularly.
- Not drinking enough water.
- Using comedogenic skin care products or makeup.

What are the treatment options?

Over-the-counter (OTC) acne medications typically rely on benzoyl peroxide, salicylic acid, and sulphur to help treat acne. Although these ingredients can help with mild breakouts, they usually aren't enough to treat hormonal acne.

Treating the underlying hormonal imbalance is the only way to clear PCOS-related acne. If you think your acne is related to PCOS, talk to your doctor or dermatologist.

Sometimes PCOS and other hormonal conditions can create too much testosterone in the body. This can increase sebum and skin cell production, leading to acne.

Not everyone with hormonal acne has high androgen levels, so your doctor will likely draw a blood sample to test your levels.

If you have PCOS-related acne, skip the OTC retinoids and see your dermatologist about prescription-strength options. They can be taken orally or applied as a topical cream or gel. The oral retinoid isotretinoin (Accutane) is the most popular option.

Retinoids make your skin extremely sensitive to the sun's UV rays, so it's vital to apply sunscreen liberally throughout the day. If your skin is left unprotected, your risk for hyperpigmentation and even skin cancer will increase.

If you opt for topical retinoids, you should only apply them in the evening. Applying them during the day can increase your risk for sun-related side effects.

Other acne treatments include:

- Reducing dairy if you feel you break out. Currently, there is no link between dairy and acne. It is usually the danger in the dose. Take note that this is very person dependent so please keep an eye on this
- Look at digestive issues like IBS and SIBO
- Look into the possibility of histamine intolerance
- Zinc
- Berberine. Please note that berberine is not safe for long term use and should be taken for no longer than 8 weeks. If you have gut issues, please be mindful that this can aggravate the problems
- DIM (diindolylmethane)
- Stress management

Please note that even with the best treatment, acne can take up to 6 months to improve. And remember that coming off the pill like Yasmin (combined pill) can cause a post pill style acne that worsens for 6 months before it gets better.

It's important to know that even the best PCOS acne treatment will do little without a good skin care routine.

Excess Facial hair

Excessive or unwanted hair that grows on a woman's body and face results from a condition called hirsutism. All women have facial and body hair, but the hair is usually very fine and light in colour.

The main difference between typical hair on a woman's body and face (often called "peach fuzz") and hair caused by hirsutism is the texture. Excessive or unwanted hair that grows on a woman's face, arms, back, or chest is usually coarse and dark. The growth pattern of hirsutism in women is associated with virilisation. Women with this condition have characteristics that are commonly associated with male hormones.

Hirsutism is excess hair in areas typically seen in men, such as the face and lower abdomen. Hypertrichosis, on the other hand, can increase hair anywhere on the body.

According to the Indian Journal of Dermatology, hirsutism affects between 5 and 10 percent of women. It tends to run in families, so you may be more likely to have unwanted hair growth if your mother, sister, or another female relative also has it.

Polycystic ovarian syndrome (PCOS) is one common cause of hirsutism. It accounts for three out of every four hirsutism cases.

Why do women grow excessive or unwanted hair?

Women develop excessive body or facial hair due to higher-than-normal levels of androgens, including testosterone. All females produce androgens, but the levels typically remain low. Certain medical conditions can cause a woman to produce too many androgens. This can drive male-pattern hair growth and other male characteristics, such as a deep voice.

Treatment for excessive or unwanted hair

- *Antiandrogen medications*: Steroidal androgens and nonsteroidal (or pure) antiandrogens can block androgen receptors and reduce androgen production from the adrenal glands, ovaries, and pituitary glands.
- *Combination birth control pills*: These pills, which have both estrogen and progesterone, may help shrink PCOS cysts. Estrogen can also help reduce excess hair. These drugs are usually a long-term solution for hirsutism. You will most likely notice improvement after three to six months of drug therapy.
- *Hair removal*: Hair removal techniques are a nonmedical way to manage excessive or unwanted hair. These are the same hair removal methods that many women use to keep their legs, bikini line, and underarms free of hair.
- *Waxing & shaving*
- *Laser hair removal*

Other natural anti-androgen treatments include:

- Zinc
- DIM (diindolylmethane)
- Micronized or natural progesterone
- Vitex or Agnus castus

Excessive or unwanted body and facial hair is a long-term challenge. Most women with diagnosed hormonal imbalances respond well to treatment, but the hair can grow back if
your hormone levels become out of sync again. If the condition makes you self-conscious, counselling and support from friends and family can help you to cope.

Myths around PCOS

1. **It's more challenging to lose weight with PCOS.**

For a very long time, there has been mention that those with PCOS have a slower BMR (lowered Basal Metabolic Rate); that's not to say it does not play a role.

"What does this mean?"
In simplest terms, it means that those with PCOS were thought to have slower metabolisms than those who do not have PCOS.

But in recent research, this opinion has changed. The first-line treatment option for overweight/obese women with PCOS is diet and lifestyle interventions; however, optimal dietary guidelines are missing.

Although many different dietary approaches have

been investigated, data on the effectiveness of very-low-calorie diets on PCOS are minimal.

A paper by Nikokavoura et al. showed after a 12-week study that the total weight loss did not differ significantly between PCOS and non-PCOS participants. Similarly, the percentage of weight loss achieved by both groups was not significantly different.

Further investigations are needed to achieve a thorough way of understanding the physiology of weight loss in PCOS. So, it's not your metabolism; it has to do with appetite regulation, binge eating, mood issues etc., that mainly cause the increase in weight amongst those who have PCOS. So, it is crucial to work on those bigger pillars rather than blaming a slower metabolism.

2. There is a perfect macro split

To understand this fully we need to know what a macro is. Macros are macronutrients. Your body needs these nutrients in larger amounts in order to function properly as macro means large. In addition, all of these nutrients provide your body with energy measured in the form of calories or kcals. There are three types of macronutrients: carbohydrates, proteins, and fats.

- Carbohydrates contain 4 kcal per gram.
- Proteins contain 4 kcal per gram.
- Fats contain 9 kcal per gram (this is roughly double the amount found in the other two macros).

- Alcohol contains 7 kcals per gram.

Along with energy, all of these macronutrients have specific roles in your body that allow you to function correctly.

So, when we are looking at your diet or anyone who has PCOS it is important to find a balance in what works for you. There is no one size fits all approach for those with PCOS or anyone else, really.

Rather than looking for a perfect macronutrient split (macro split) why not focus on getting decent levels of protein with each meal, alongside fats, carbs (wholegrain where possible), veggies and fruit to help manage PCOS. This is not only for PCOS but for everyone.

3. You can't have carbohydrates

Carbs have a bad reputation for a very long time but particularly with those with PCOS. For those with the Insulin resistant form of PCOS, you must monitor your carb intake. This does not mean that you should go full Keto (The ketogenic diet is a high-fat, adequate-protein, low-carbohydrate diet that in medicine is used mainly to treat hard-to-control epilepsy in children)

For those with Insulin resistant PCOS, your body may try to pump out high levels of insulin to keep your blood sugar levels normal. Too-high levels of insulin can cause your ovaries to produce more androgens, such as testosterone.

Insulin resistance may also be caused by having a body mass index above the normal range. Insulin resistance can make it harder to lose weight, which is why women with PCOS often experience this issue.

A diet high in refined carbohydrates, such as starchy and sugary foods, can make insulin resistance and weight loss more difficult to control. This does not mean cutting them out completely; it means being a bit more cautious than someone who may not have Insulin Resistant PCOS.

Where possible, aim for whole grain, high fibre, higher protein and regular meals will help you a lot more than cutting out an entire food group.

PCOS & IBS

It's so important first to define what IBS is. Irritable bowel syndrome (IBS) is a common condition that affects the digestive system. It causes symptoms like stomach cramps, bloating, diarrhoea and constipation. These tend to come and go over time and can last for days, weeks or months at a time. It's usually a lifelong problem. Some of the symptoms include Constipation; Abdominal pain & Diarrhoea.

If you have PCOS, you may also experience IBS. The two conditions may be linked in several ways.

So, what's the connection?

Excess hormones

PCOS is marked by excess levels of luteinizing hormone (LH) and follicle-stimulating hormone (FSH), which are involved in ovulation. As a result, ovulation does not occur, leading to irregular menstrual periods.

High levels of these hormones can also cause IBS. According to 2020 entitled Sex-Gender Differences in Irritable Bowel Syndrome, excess LH and FSH can delay food movement in the digestive tract, resulting in constipation.

In the same study, the authors noted that women are twice as likely to have IBS compared with people who are assigned male at birth. Therefore, being a woman increases your risk of having both conditions.

Although it's unclear why the condition is more common in women, it's thought to be related to:

- *Sex hormones.* Estrogen and progesterone, two female sex hormones, may cause constipation by slowing down intestinal muscle contractions. These hormones fluctuate during menstruation, which can cause diarrhoea. Remember the only way for women to get rid of the old cycle is to go to the bathroom.
- *Higher pain perception.* Female sex hormones also increase the perception of pain. Women are more likely to feel stomach cramps and discomfort due to bowel issues.

- *Higher stress levels.* Female sex hormones also increase your susceptibility to stress, which can lead to IBS symptoms. Having PCOS can increase stress levels.

Inflammation

PCOS and IBS may be linked via inflammation. According to a 2019 study, PCOS causes chronic inflammation. This can lead to inflammatory conditions like type 2 diabetes and heart disease. Inflammation can also play a role in the development of IBS.

Symptoms of PCOS and IBS

It's very important to understand the common symptoms between PCOS and IBS and realise the symptoms of PCOS and IBS can vary greatly.

Common PCOS symptoms include:

- Irregular periods
- Acne
- Oily skin
- Thinning hair
- Excess face and body hair
- Ovarian cysts
- large ovaries
- Skin darkening
- Thick skin patches
- Trouble getting pregnant
- Unexplained weight gain

Typical IBS symptoms include:

- Abdominal pain
- Bowel changes
- Diarrhoea, constipation, or both
- Bloating
- Feeling like you have not finished passing stool
- Whitish mucus in stool

If you think you have PCOS and IBS, talk with a primary care doctor.
You should also see a doctor if you have any of the following:

- Irregular or no periods
- Unexplained weight gain
- Unexplained bowel changes
- Persistent bloating
- Difficulty getting pregnant

If your primary care doctor thinks you have PCOS and IBS, they'll refer you to a gynaecologist and gastroenterologist. A gynaecologist specialises in the female reproductive system, while a gastroenterologist specialises in the digestive system.

You can also mention your symptoms at your yearly gynaecologist appointment. Since digestive symptoms are often associated with PCOS and other reproductive disorders, it's important to tell your gynaecologist about them.

Also, if you think you have one condition but not the other, you should still see a doctor. Please go back to look at the diagnosis part of this chapter on how to get a Diagnosis.

Treatment

The first line of treatment involves lifestyle changes, followed by medication.

- *Dietary changes.* Eating a nutrient-rich, balanced diet as often as possible can ease some symptoms of PCOS. If you also have IBS, it may help to eat more fibre, avoid or limit gluten, or follow a low FODMAP diet.
- *Stress management.* Since stress plays a role in both conditions, your doctor will recommend stress relief. This may include exercise, adequate sleep, or therapy.
- *Stress management.* Since stress plays a role in both conditions, your doctor will recommend stress relief. This may include exercise, adequate sleep, or therapy.
- *Medication.* Your doctor may prescribe medication for PCOS symptoms like irregular periods, excess hair growth, and fertility issues. They may also prescribe IBS medications for diarrhoea, constipation, or abdominal pain.

It's worth noting that taking some medications for one condition might negatively affect the other. So please make your medical professional aware of everything that you are on during the consultation.

For instance, PCOS increases your risk for diabetes. Your doctor might recommend metformin, which lowers your blood sugar levels. But metformin may have side effects like diarrhoea, constipation, and gas, which can worsen IBS symptoms and may worsen insulin resistance.

Antidepressants, which may be used to ease IBS symptoms, may be recommended. That's because depression may contribute to IBS. However, using antidepressants for a long time may be linked to an increase in your risk for diabetes, which is also higher with PCOS.

If you have both conditions, it's important to communicate with your healthcare professional continually. Keeping the lines of communication open will help you get to the root and live a freer life.

Managing IBS

Since there's no cure for either condition, living with PCOS and IBS depends on effective disease management.

This primarily involves lifestyle changes, such as:

- Staying as physically active as possible
- Eating a nutrient-rich, balanced diet as often as possible
- Managing stress, anxiety, and depression
- Avoiding IBS triggers

Understandably, it can be challenging to adopt specific lifestyle changes. Do not hesitate to ask your doctors for tips or guidance.
Disease management is crucial for PCOS, and for the best advice, attend your regular check-ups, so

your doctor can monitor your symptoms and offer personalised advice.

The link?

PCOS and IBS might be connected in several ways. PCOS is marked by high ovarian hormones, which can affect how your bowels work. Both conditions also involve inflammation. What's more, IBS is more common in women than men.

See a primary care doctor if you think you have PCOS and/or IBS. They may refer you to a gynaecologist and gastroenterologist for further evaluation.

Treatment for PCOS and IBS mainly involves lifestyle changes, which can help you find relief and manage both conditions.

Talking to your doctor

Talking to your doctor and having a strong relationship with your medical professional is essential in managing your PCOS. This can be an uneasy time for you, but it can also be a place of discovery and getting to the root cause can provide you with the opportunity to live the life you ultimately want.

It is important to be prepared for your meetings with your doctor so that they can put you at ease and answer anything you are unsure of.
Some of the questions that you could ask include:

- What is your treatment plan for my PCOS?
- That type of PCOS do I have?
- Is my thyroid gland healthy and functioning normally?
- Am I at risk for diabetes?
- How are my cholesterol levels?
- Are there any other health concerns that I should be aware of?
- Can I get pregnant?
- Can I get a full hormone screen?
- What is the plan to re-diagnose? (This may be where you mention the DUTCH Test that was mentioned earlier in the chapter)
- What is the next step?

Please remember you are fully entitled to have your hormones screened. Please make sure that you get a copy of the results if the practitioner does not go through them with you. Remember it is your body, and you have full right to understand how it works and how to manage it to live the life you wish.

Prolactin

Prolactin is another important element in PCOS and the overall hormone health of a woman's body.

High Prolactin:

The pituitary gland produces prolactin in the brain. It's also known as PRL or lactogenic hormone. Prolactin is mainly used to help women produce milk after childbirth. Too much prolactin inhibits ovulation.

Severely elevated prolactin levels are a serious

medical condition that can stop periods completely.

Mildly elevated prolactin can cause other issues, too; some of these include irregular periods, breast pain, loss of libido and can also cause androgen excess.

High prolactin can be identified with a blood test. The test can also rule out other pituitary gland or hypothalamus problems.

A prolactin test is just like a blood test. It takes a few minutes at your doctor's office or in a lab. You don't need to prepare for it. The sample is typically collected three to four hours after waking up in the morning. Blood is drawn from a vein in your arm. There's very little pain. You may only feel a slight pinch when the needle goes in and some mild soreness afterwards.

Some birth control pills, high blood pressure drugs, or antidepressants can affect the test results. Tell your doctor about any medications you're taking before the test is done. Sleeping problems, high stress levels, and strenuous exercise before the test can also influence the results.

What are normal results?

Normal results usually look like the following (ng/mL = nanograms per millilitre):

Women who are not pregnant   < 25 ng/mL
Women who are pregnant   34 to 386 ng/mL

What do high levels mean?

A reading greater than 1000 mIU/L or 50ng/mL is usually the reading for someone with higher prolactin levels.

High levels of prolactin are normal during pregnancy and after childbirth during nursing.

However, hyperprolactinemia can also be caused by anorexia nervosa, liver disease, kidney disease, and hypothyroidism. Hypothyroidism can cause enlargement of the pituitary gland, which is treatable with thyroid hormone replacement therapy.

Pituitary tumours can also cause high levels of prolactin. These tumours can be treated medically or surgically.

Certain medications can cause high prolactin levels. Psychiatric drugs such as risperidone and haloperidol can increase your levels. Metoclopramide can also raise your prolactin levels. This medication is normally used to treat acid reflux or nausea caused by cancer drugs.

Some everyday stressors can also raise prolactin levels. These stressors include low blood sugar, strenuous exercise activities, and even mild forms of discomfort. If you find out that your prolactin levels are high, you may need to find ways to reduce your stress and keep your blood sugar at consistent levels.

Moderately high prolactin:

A reading greater than 480 mIU/L or 23ng/mL is usually the reading for someone with moderately high prolactin levels. This can be caused by a prolactinoma, thyroid disease, alcohol, some medications such as hormonal birth control. This requires a medical diagnosis.

Mildly high prolactin

A reading greater than 480 mIU/L or 23ng/mL is usually the reading for someone with mildly high prolactin levels. A single test cannot diagnose this. It can be elevated by sex, exercise, alcohol, sleep, dehydration, stress, luteal phase, mild thyroid disease or hormonal birth control.

Prolactin and fertility

In some cases, high prolactin levels can lead to infertility. High prolactin levels can interrupt the normal production of the hormones estrogen and progesterone. This can cause the ovaries to release eggs irregularly or stop altogether.

Medications and other prolactinoma treatments help restore fertility in most women. If you find out you have high prolactin levels or prolactinoma tumours, talk to your doctor right away about treatments. You can also ask about removing or reducing tumours.

Treatment for high prolactin levels

Once your doctor has ruled out a medical explanation for your high prolactin, you can consider using natural treatments.

Treatment for high prolactin levels include:

- changing your diet and keeping your stress levels down
- stopping high-intensity workouts or activities that overwhelm you
- Reducing alcohol (beer can stimulate prolactin)
- Introduce Yoga or meditation into your life
- Vitex (if you are on antidepressant medication, please consult with doctor first)
- Vitamin E supplements (may decrease prolactin in instances of uraemia, but there is currently no evidence in otherwise healthy controls)
- Mucuna or L-DOPA ingestion
- Vitamin B6 (300mg x2 per day)

Sometimes there's no specific cause for your high prolactin levels. This is known as idiopathic hyperprolactinemia. It usually goes away without treatment after several months. If your prolactin levels do not go down, your doctor will likely prescribe medication. Please link in with your medical professional.

Conclusion

PCOS does not mean your life has to be uncomfortable or that you can't live a normal life.

If you find out what type of PCOS that you have this will guide you in how you should manage your symptoms.

Losing weight can help manage PCOS, but an important caveat is that not everyone with PCOS is overweight so this may not be an option for those individuals.

Losing weight is possible but it may mean being a little more patient. Please work with a Dietitian or a Nutritionist to help you through this. Nutritionally higher protein, moderate carbs and fats intake will benefit you massively.

Mental health plays a massive role with PCOS alongside fertility and digestive issues. Please be aware it can take longer to conceive with PCOS so please work with a doctor or someone to guide you on these.

PCOS is not a mindset, it is a very common condition and it can be managed. You can live the life you want once you understand your symptoms.

Chapter 6 - Endometriosis

What is Endometriosis?

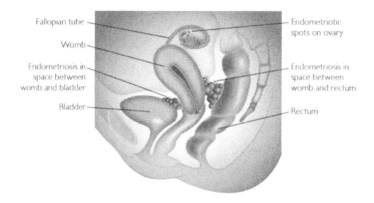

Endometriosis is a disorder in which tissue similar to the tissue that forms the lining of your uterus grows outside of your uterine cavity. Endometriosis occurs when endometrial tissue grows on your ovaries, bowel, and tissues lining your pelvis. It's unusual for endometrial tissue to spread beyond your pelvic region, but it's not impossible.

The lining of your uterus is called the endometrium. Endometriosis is a common gynaecological condition, affecting up to 10 percent of women.

Endometriosis occurs when endometrial tissue grows on your ovaries, bowel, and tissues lining your pelvis. It's unusual for endometrial tissue to spread beyond your pelvic region, but it's not impossible.

The hormonal changes of your menstrual cycle

affect the misplaced endometrial tissue, causing the area to become inflamed and painful. This can be extremely painful for some women. This means the tissue will grow, thicken, and break down. Over time, the tissue that has broken down has nowhere to go and becomes trapped in your pelvis.

This tissue trapped in your pelvis can cause:

- Irritation
- Scar formation
- Adhesions (in which tissue binds your pelvic organs together)
- Severe pain during your periods
- Fertility problems

At present the evidence is relatively low compared to that of PCOS. A lot more research is needed to fully understand the full impact of Endometriosis on someone's life.

Although the exact cause of Endometriosis is not certain, possible explanations include:

- Retrograde menstruation. In retrograde menstruation, menstrual blood containing endometrial cells flows back through the fallopian tubes and into the pelvic cavity instead of out of the body. These endometrial cells stick to the pelvic walls and surfaces of pelvic organs, where they grow and continue to thicken and bleed over the course of each menstrual cycle.
- Transformation of peritoneal cells.

- Embryonic cell transformation. Hormones such as estrogen may transform embryonic cells — cells in the earliest stages of development — into endometrial-like cell implants during puberty.
- Surgical scar implantation.
- Endometrial cell transport.
- Immune system disorder. A problem with the immune system may make the body unable to recognize and destroy endometrial-like tissue that's growing outside the uterus.

As research is still quite new more research is needed but the general consensus is caused by immune dysfunction. Endometriosis shares some similarities with the likes of lupus and rheumatoid arthritis.

There is also a strong genetic component to Endometriosis. If someone in your family like your mother or your sister has Endometriosis, then there is a high possibility that you will develop it yourself.

You're not alone if you have this disorder.

Endometriosis symptoms

The symptoms of Endometriosis vary. Some women experience mild symptoms, but others can have moderate to severe symptoms. The severity of your pain doesn't indicate the degree or stage of the condition. You may have a mild form of the disease yet experience agonizing pain. It's also possible to have a severe form and have very little discomfort.

Pelvic pain is the most common symptom of Endometriosis. You may also have the following symptoms:

- painful periods
- pain in the lower abdomen before and during menstruation
- cramps one or two weeks around menstruation
- heavy menstrual bleeding or bleeding between periods
- infertility
- pain following sexual intercourse
- discomfort with bowel movements
- lower back pain that may occur at any time during your menstrual cycle

You may also have no symptoms.

It's important that you get regular gynaecological exams, which will allow your gynaecologist to monitor any changes. This is particularly important if you have two or more symptoms.

Diagnosis of Endometriosis

The symptoms of Endometriosis can be similar to the symptoms of other conditions, such as ovarian cysts and pelvic inflammatory disease. Treating your pain requires an accurate diagnosis. Your doctor will perform one or more of the following tests:

Detailed history

Your doctor will note your symptoms and personal or family history of Endometriosis. A general health assessment may also be performed to determine if there are any other signs of a long-term disorder.

Physical exam

During a pelvic exam, your doctor will manually feel your abdomen for cysts or scars behind the uterus.

Ultrasound

Your doctor may use a transvaginal ultrasound or an abdominal ultrasound. In a transvaginal ultrasound, a transducer is inserted into your vagina.

A pelvic ultrasound cannot usually detect Endometriosis lesions, but it can sometimes detect more serious forms or Endometriosis. It is important to note that Endometriosis cannot be ruled out by an ultrasound.

Endometriosis is a chronic condition with no cure.
We don't understand what causes it yet.
But this doesn't mean the condition has to impact your daily life.

Endometriosis treatment

Understandably, you want quick relief from pain and other symptoms of Endometriosis. This condition can disrupt your life if it's left untreated.

Endometriosis has no cure, but its symptoms can be managed.

Medical and surgical options are available to help reduce your symptoms and manage any potential complications. Your doctor may first try conservative treatments. They may then recommend surgery if your condition doesn't improve. Please consult with a doctor or a dietician if you think you may suffer from Endometriosis.

Pain medications

You can try over-the-counter pain medications such as ibuprofen, but these aren't effective in all cases. Please consult with a medical professional to get medication.

Some of the options include Hormone Therapy, Contraceptives, Medroxyprogesterone (Depo-Provera) injection, Gonadotropin-releasing hormone (GnRH) agonists and antagonists, Danazol and there are other drugs are being studied that may improve symptoms and slow disease progress.

There are also other options available including Conservative surgery, Laparoscopy, and as a Last-resort surgery a hysterectomy.

Laparoscopy

The only certain method for identifying Endometriosis is by viewing it directly. This is done by a minor surgical procedure known as a laparoscopy. Once diagnosed, the tissue can be removed in the same procedure. It may seem to be a little outdated but it is currently the only method of diagnosis.

The success of the surgery will depend on the skill and training of the surgeon and whether he or she manages to remove all of the lesions. There is some research that a surgery called an excision surgery is more successful in the long term. More research is needed on this.

Like with anything there can be downsides to surgery and these include the fact that it requires general anaesthetic and recovery. Another important downside is that it can cause adhesions or scar tissue, which can then cause pain.

As mentioned before surgery does not cure Endometriosis. The rate of recurrence following surgery is 21% after two years and 40-50% after five years. This can ultimately lead to more surgeries. From research the medical solution is to give hormone suppressing drugs to try and prevent this.

Research on Endometriosis is forever evolving and research is looking into a simple test that would use a bio marker found in blood, saliva, urine, menstrual blood or the uterine lining. This could lead to a diagnosis being made through a non-invasive test. This is at the very early stages so this may take time to evolve into something that can be further used for diagnosis.

Surgery is currently the primary conventional treatment. We need to be aware that surgery does not cure Endometriosis. It can relieve pain and may improve fertility.

Rarely, your doctor may recommend a total hysterectomy as a last resort if your condition doesn't improve with other treatments. It is important that you discuss all of your options with your doctor.

Risk factors

Endometriosis usually develops years after the start of your menstrual cycle. This condition can be painful but understanding the risk factors can help you determine whether you're susceptible to this condition and when you should talk to your doctor.

- *Age* - Women of all ages are at risk for Endometriosis. It usually affects women between the ages of 25 and 40, but symptoms can begin at puberty.
- *Family history* - Talk to your doctor if you have a family member who has Endometriosis. You may have a higher risk of developing the disease.
- *Pregnancy history* - Pregnancy may temporarily decrease the symptoms of Endometriosis. Women who haven't had children run a greater risk of developing the disorder. However, Endometriosis can still occur in women who've had children. This supports the understanding that hormones influence the development and progress of the condition.
- *Menstrual history* - Talk to your doctor if you have problems regarding your period. These

issues can include shorter cycles, heavier and longer periods, or menstruation that starts at a young age. These factors may place you at higher risk.

Diet and Lifestyle for Endometriosis

Endometriosis is a multifactorial disease, and we still don't fully understand its pathogenesis.

So, we can't really quantify the effect of diet, but there are a few things that you can make sure is to try include in your diet including:

- Anti-Inflammatory/ Anti - Oxidant Foods including Omega 3&6 Fatty Acids (Fatty Fish, Flaxseed, Soy beans, Nuts, Seeds)
- Lots of fruits and veggies
- Wholegrains
- Eggs, Peanuts (sources of Pea)
- Cruciferous Veggies (Brussel Sprouts, just be mindful of Broccoli as some women can have flare ups after consumption)
- Wide variety of food (Vitamins, Minerals & Antioxidants)
- Please be mindful of Alcohol Consumption
- Please be mindful of Trans Fats (Margarine, Processed food etc)
- Dairy - Sometimes a dairy free diet is suggested as a good option but a large study (120,706 samples) found quite the opposite. The study found that women with high dairy intake vs low have a 17% reduced risk for Endometriosis. As dairy intake increases the risk of Endometriosis decreases. Total dairy

intake of >21 servings/ week or average of 3 servings/ day significantly reduced the risk of Endometriosis by 13% compared to women with no/ low dairy intake.

Reducing foods like the ones listed above have some shown evidence to help manage symptoms but more evidence is needed.

Supplements that might help

- Omega 3/6 (if not regularly in your diet)
- Vitamin D (if not regularly exposed to sufficient sunshine)
- Iron as Iron levels will need to be checked as woman who have Endometriosis may be anaemic
- DIM (more evidence is needed on this)
- Zinc
- B- Vitamins
- N-acetyl cysteine (NAC) has shown to reduce the size of cysts, reduction in pain
- Curcumin (Turmeric) - is known for having anti-inflammatory properties, which was confirmed in a 2009 review. A further 2013 study suggested that curcumin may help with Endometriosis by reducing estradiol production.
- Ashwagandha - A 2014 review found that clinically significant reductions in stress resulted from treatment with the herb ashwagandha. Another study in 2006 found that women with advanced Endometriosis had significantly higher levels of cortisol, a hormone involved in stress response. And as

we know stress management plays a huge role in managing Endometriosis.

More research is needed on supplementation for Endometriosis. Please do not take all of these supplements together. Consider taking Zinc, turmeric and NAC.

The first point of call should be to seek a referral to a gynaecologist and talk through all of the options regarding the next step.

Training with Endometriosis

Some women with Endometriosis can become generally weakened from the cycle of inflammation, stress and pain. Strength training becomes especially important in order to build strength through all the muscle groups, especially the weakened muscles. Aiming for three weight sessions per week is a safe place to start.

<u>Pelvic Floor exercises</u>

In most women, pelvic floor engagement is recommended during the exhale breath. However, in women with hypertonic pelvic floor muscles, cueing for pelvic floor engagement can cause more pain and discomfort. Therefore, in these circumstances, pelvic floor relaxation is encouraged.

Instead of doing "Kegels" or pelvic floor lifts, women with hypertonic pelvic floor muscles need to do "reverse Kegels" or pelvic floor drops.

<u>Physio</u>

Physiotherapy can also be very beneficial for adhesions, pain and pelvic floor dysfunction.

<u>Yoga</u>

It is also important for women who have Endometriosis to stretch the muscles around their hips, pelvis, back and abdomen. Incorporating yoga into your exercise habits, or having a diligent stretch routine during your warmup and cool-down that flows through these muscles on the days when your strength training, are both useful ways of addressing this.

Keep in mind that the connective tissue in the pelvic floor and in the abdomen can become tight due to scarring and adhesions. Therefore, exercises that shorten these muscle groups such as crunches and sit-ups may not be ideal. Exercises that strengthen the muscles in these areas in an elongated position would be more justified.

If you are having flare ups, please try to avoid the likes of running, high intensity workouts and focus on light exercise including walking, yoga or meditations. Every woman will be different so it is important to understand your body.

Fertility and Endometriosis

Having issues with fertility is a serious complication of Endometriosis. Most treatments for Endometriosis aim to prevent ovulation. One example is taking birth control pills. When you're trying to get pregnant, you'll stop taking these treatments. Fertility in general can unfortunately also be affected by Endometriosis.

Women with milder forms may be able to conceive and carry a baby to term. According to the Mayo Clinic, about 30% – 40% of women with Endometriosis have trouble getting pregnant. A 2014 review of studies found that 2 to 10 percent of couples living with Endometriosis succeeded in becoming pregnant versus 15 to 20 percent of couples without Endometriosis as a complication.

Fertility issues due to Endometriosis can be related to several causes. The first is if Endometriosis affects the ovaries and/or fallopian tubes.

In order to get pregnant an egg must travel from the ovary, past the fallopian tube, and to the uterus for fertilization before implantation into the uterine lining. If a woman has Endometriosis in her fallopian tube lining, the tissue may keep the egg from traveling to the uterus.

It's also possible that Endometriosis could damage an egg or a sperm. While doctors don't know exactly why this occurs, a theory is that Endometriosis causes greater levels of inflammation in the body. More research is needed on this to provide the full picture.

When to see a doctor?

Some doctors may recommend seeing a fertility specialist before you start trying to become pregnant.

A fertility specialist may conduct blood tests, such as an anti-Mullerian hormone (AMH) test. This test reflects your remaining egg supply. Another term for egg supply is "ovarian reserve."

Surgical Endometriosis treatments can reduce your ovarian reserve, so you may want to consider this test when thinking about Endometriosis treatments.

The only way to truly diagnose Endometriosis is surgery to identify areas where endometrium-like tissue is present. But these surgeries could potentially result in scarring that may affect fertility. This is usually minor, but talk with your doctor about risks and benefits.

Guidance for endometriosis-related infertility

If you have been trying for over 6 months please talk to your doctor. A doctor will be able to go through the various options for you. They will link in with a fertility specialist to determine what is going on and the severity of your Endometriosis.

Some of the treatments that are on the table for Endometriosis fertility issues include:

- *Freezing your eggs*: Endometriosis can affect your ovarian reserve, so some doctors may recommend preserving your eggs now in case you wish to become pregnant later. This option can be costly, and isn't usually covered by insurance so this will need to be taken into account.

- *Superovulation and intrauterine insemination (SO-IUI):* This is an option for those who have normal fallopian tubes, mild Endometriosis, and whose partner has sperm with no fertility issues.
- *A doctor can prescribe fertility medications such as Clomiphene.* These medications help to produce two to three mature eggs. A doctor may also prescribe progestin injections.
- A person trying to get pregnant may regularly undergo ultrasounds to ensure the eggs are at their most mature. When the eggs are ready, a doctor will insert a partner's collected sperm.
- *In vitro fertilization (IVF):* This treatment involves extracting an egg from you and sperm from your partner. The egg is then fertilized outside the body and implanted into the uterus.

The success rates of IVF for those with Endometriosis are about half of the success rates of those with other reasons for fertility issues. But many people with Endometriosis have successfully gotten pregnant thanks to IVF treatments. So, there is still hope.

IVF is often recommended for people with moderate to severe Endometriosis, or for those whose bodies haven't responded to other treatments.

What can be done to improve your chances of conceiving with Endometriosis?

Currently, there's no evidence that medication can improve a person's chances of getting pregnant with Endometriosis. But doctors may prescribe medications, such as progestins, to increase the amount of pregnancy hormones in the body.

It's also important to live as healthy a lifestyle as possible when you have Endometriosis and are trying to get pregnant. This can reduce inflammation in your body and prepare it to help your baby grow and thrive throughout a healthy pregnancy.

<u>What can be done?</u>

- Maintaining a healthy-for-you weight
- Mediterranean diet
- Eating nutrient-dense foods rich in fruits, vegetables, whole grains, and lean proteins
- Engaging in moderate exercise on a daily basis (examples include walking, lifting weights, and participating in an exercise class)

Keep in mind that age can be a factor for anyone wishing to get pregnant. Higher fertility rates are associated with younger age. Women ages 35 and older are at an increased risk for both fertility issues and miscarriage than younger women.

You might want to consider having children sooner rather than later if you've been diagnosed with Endometriosis and you want children. Your symptoms may worsen over time, which can make it difficult to conceive on your own. You'll need to be assessed by your doctor before and during pregnancy.

Even if fertility isn't a concern, managing chronic pain can be difficult. Depression, anxiety, and other mental issues aren't uncommon. Talk to your doctor about ways to deal with these side effects. Joining a support group could be a great option too.

The good news is that there are many people living with Endometriosis who conceive and ultimately deliver a healthy baby. The key is to start discussing your conception options, sometimes even before you think about getting pregnant.

When you're trying to get pregnant, talk with your doctor if you haven't conceived after 6 months of trying.

Can you have PCOS and Endometriosis?

You can have Endometriosis and PCOS at the same time. In fact, a 2015 study found that women with PCOS are more likely to be diagnosed with Endometriosis.

Another 2014 study determined that there's a strong link between Endometriosis and PCOS with pelvic pain and/or trouble getting pregnant.

According to an older 2011 study, the high levels of androgens and insulin in PCOS could indirectly increase estradiol. This may increase the risk of

Endometriosis.

Diagnosing Endometriosis vs. PCOS

Your doctor will use several tests to determine if you have Endometriosis, PCOS, or both.

Generally, your doctor will use the tests mentioned earlier in the chapter to see if you have symptoms like irregular periods. But if you don't have symptoms, you may receive a diagnosis while you're being treated for something else. Here is a quick list of the tests that could be used:

- Detailed look into medical history
- Physical exam
- Ultrasound (It is important to note that Endometriosis cannot be ruled out by an ultrasound)

Does treatment differ for PCOS and Endometriosis

Both conditions are treated with various forms of medication and surgery.

Endometriosis

Treatment focuses on reducing estrogen and pain. Options include:

- Medication for estrogen: Medication, like birth control, can help reduce estrogen and regulate growth of endometrial tissue.

- Pain medication: Over-the-counter pain medication may provide relief.
- Surgical removal of tissue: A surgeon removes endometrial tissue growth.
- Hysterectomy: Hysterectomy, or removal of the uterus, may be recommended if you're not trying to conceive.
- Lifestyle changes: A balanced, nutrient-rich diet can help manage your symptoms.
- Stress and sleep management

PCOS

Please see the PCOS chapter on this for more information. Treatments include:

- Medication: Your doctor should provide you with all of the various options for this.
- Acne or hair medication: These drugs help manage acne or excess hair growth.
- Laparoscopic ovarian drilling: If ovulation drugs don't help, your doctor might recommend this surgery. It destroys the androgen-releasing tissue in the ovaries.
- Weight management: A healthy diet and regular exercise could help you lose weight, which may manage your symptoms. Weight loss will not cure PCOS it may just make your life easier as you
- Wholesome balanced diet
- Stress and sleep management

With Endometriosis, uterine tissue grows in other parts of the body, causing pain and infertility. It's linked to high estrogen levels, so treatment focuses on reducing estrogen and pain.

PCOS, on the other hand, is due to high levels of androgens. It may cause infertility and ovarian cysts.

Endometriosis and PCOS are common. It's also possible to have both at the same time. If you have abnormal periods or difficulty conceiving, visit your gynaecologist.

Gut health and Endometriosis

Endometriosis can have a huge impact on your gut. It's important to remember that although we don't know why Endometriosis happens, it's both an inflammatory disease as well as a disease dependent on estrogen.

Up to 90% of women with Endometriosis also experience bowel symptoms. The effects of an over-excited uterus can include painful periods, ongoing and excessive abdominal pain, nausea, fatigue and fertility issues. On top of these unwanted symptoms, women with Endometriosis are more likely to experience symptoms of IBS, which can make for a very unhappy abdomen.

From an anatomical perspective, it makes sense that what's going on in your small and large intestine, may influence the symptoms in your uterus and ovaries, and vice versa. They are sitting right next to one another after all. And when you have all that machinery crammed in together, it can sometimes be difficult to determine what's causing what.

Your gastrointestinal (GI) tract pushes food and poo along the tube by using the muscles that line the tract. The muscles squeeze and release in a wave movement that's called peristalsis

In some cases, endometrial lesions around the uterus and bowel can cause excessive pain and discomfort as your GI tract squeezes food and poo along with this wave.

Equally, if you have a blockage in the large intestine due to constipation, or you have a build-up of gas in the large intestine, this can put pressure on the uterus and ovaries, exacerbating the pain and discomfort of Endometriosis.

For some women, endometrial cells can even intrude into the bowel, which can cause inflammation, obstruction of the bowel and even micro-haemorrhages.

So, from this perspective, Endometriosis and gut health are already closely linked purely due to their proximity, and managing GI symptoms could help manage Endo symptoms.

Gut microbes and Estrogen

Over the past few decades, we have learnt more and more about the bacteria in our gut and the role that they play in our bowel health, immunity and brain health. Interestingly, the bacteria in our gut can also influence your hormones, including estrogen.

Because estrogen contributes to the growth of endometrial tissue, there is an emerging theory that changes to your gut microbes may impact Endometriosis.

Within the gut, there is a collection of bacteria which are able to process estrogen and modulate the body's estrogen levels. This group of bacteria is collectively called the estrobolome.

Estrogen is made by the ovaries, adrenal glands and fat cells in the body, it then travels around our body in the bloodstream. Then it is metabolised and changed in the liver before being eliminated through our urine or the bile that's being excreted in our poo.

Amazingly, the estrobolome bacteria can change these eliminated estrogens back into their original shape, allowing them to be reabsorbed from the gut, back into the bloodstream, thereby increasing estrogen in the blood.

There are lots of things that might affect the balance of your estrobolome, including:

- Age
- Ethnicity
- Genetics
- Diet
- Alcohol
- Antibiotic use
- Gut microbes and inflammation

There is some evidence to suggest that your

bacteria (microbiome) contribute to, or is involved in, the regulation of inflammatory factors, which may influence endometrial lesion development.

Your bacteria break down a whole range of chemicals from your food including fibre and resistant starches. The bacteria then create by-products or metabolites, which are really a fancy way of saying 'bacteria poo'.

Your body absorbs the metabolites (bacteria poo) and then those chemicals affect your pathways of your immune system, particularly inflammatory markers. This can signal more or less inflammation, depending on the bacteria and the metabolite.

The exact pathway of how particular bacteria influence inflammation in Endometriosis is not yet clear, but it's an emerging area of research.

So, what do we do?

As you can see, there are lots of ways that Endometriosis might be affected by gut health and vice versa. But, given this is all new and emerging knowledge, what do we do with it?

We can't yet make recommendations on taking a particular probiotic or eating particular foods to help endo, but we can take steps to support our gut health and manage gut symptoms, which may help in the management of Endometriosis.

Here's how to support a healthy gut:

1. *Fibre* - Think veggies and fruit.
2. *Water* - H2O is essential for keeping everything moving through your gut. Reducing the risk of constipation helps to reduce pressure within your abdominal cavity, which can lessen the pressure on endometrial lesions and help to manage pain.
3. *Physical activity* - Moving your body helps to stimulate the muscles of the bowel to push things through, which again helps with constipation.
4. *Sleep* - There is growing evidence that the quality and duration of our sleep can affect gut bacteria. Getting more sleep-in total supports a greater diversity of gut bacteria, and waking during the night appears to reduce this diversity. Research has shown 7-9 hours is a decent number to aim for.

How to manage gut symptoms

If you are suffering from IBS style symptoms in the context of Endometriosis, the aim may be to minimise the impact of gut symptoms on your Endometriosis symptoms. These are some ways you can do it:

- *Investigate FODMAPs* - A FODMAP intolerance is a common contributor to IBS. FODMAP's are fermentable carbohydrates that our bacteria feed off and produce lots of gas. This gas can cause bloating and changes to stool consistency, all of which

create more pressure and discomfort in the abdomen, where you may have endometrial lesions. Trialling a low FODMAP elimination diet with a dietitian can help you better understand how to avoid triggering foods and feel better.
- *Muscle relaxants* - There is some evidence that these herbal remedies may have an antispasmodic effect, meaning that they help to reduce the spasm of your gastrointestinal muscles, which is what causes cramping and pain:
    - Peppermint Oil
    - Ginger
    - Chamomile

However, I would recommend speaking to your GP or a health professional before commencing a new medication, even an over the counter one. Probiotics need to be tailored to the individual so please don't grab any type in a shop.

Menopause and Endometriosis

The interesting thing is that your symptoms will improve after menopause. The reasons for symptoms improving after menopause is due to the endometrial tissue needing the hormone estrogen to grow. When you go through menopause naturally, your ovaries produce less estrogen. And if you have surgery and your ovaries are removed, you no longer produce as much estrogen. As a result, your symptoms may lessen.

If symptoms continue after menopause please consult with your doctor and they may suggest surgery.

Conclusion

Endometriosis is a chronic condition with no cure. We don't understand what causes it yet.

But this doesn't mean the condition has to impact your daily life. Effective treatments are available to manage pain and fertility issues, such as medications, hormone therapy, and surgery. The symptoms of Endometriosis usually improve after menopause but this isn't the case for everybody.

You can still exercise with Endometriosis and it is so important to pick the right one at the right time. Managing your exercise around various symptoms will save you so much heartache if you know what type works for you or even when you need to rest.

Sleep and stress play a huge factor in how your symptoms affect your body. Knowing that you are not alone should really help you to live the life that you want.

Chapter 7 - Pre and Post Natal Training and Nutrition

Having kids is one of the most amazing things that someone goes through. The body can go through many changes at different stages, so I think this is incredibly important to understand how to train and eat at various stages of the pregnancy.

Pregnancy - How does it happen?

Pregnancy occurs when a sperm fertilizes an egg after it's released from the ovary during ovulation.

The fertilized egg then travels down into the uterus, where implantation occurs.

A successful implantation results in pregnancy. On average, a full-term pregnancy lasts 40 weeks. Many factors can affect a pregnancy. Women who receive an early pregnancy diagnosis and prenatal care are more likely to experience a healthy pregnancy and give birth to a healthy baby.

Before getting pregnant, achieving an ideal weight before conception provides better health outcomes for both mother and baby. This is not to say that you can't or shouldn't conceive if outside of this BMI.

Try not to get too caught up on the BMI marker as I have seen clients get pregnant and have amazing pregnancies at a higher weight.

Getting Pregnant

After you've made the decision to have a baby, many women try to do everything they can to conceive during their next cycle. But it's important to remember that getting pregnant can take time.

This is where flashbacks of your Sexual Education class come back in, and your teacher probably made it sound like you can get pregnant any time you have sex. But in truth, it's a little more complicated.

Each month, there are a series of hormonal changes in your body that cause an immature egg in the ovary to grow and mature. Every woman's cycle is different. This process takes about two weeks on average, beginning with a woman's menstrual period.

Once the egg is mature, it's released from the ovary in a process known as ovulation. The egg then travels down the fallopian tube toward the uterus. The egg is only viable for about 24 hours once released.

If the egg is fertilized by a sperm cell during this time frame, the fertilized egg will keep travelling down toward the uterus. It will then implant into the uterine lining.

The key is to have sex on the days before and during ovulation. That way, the sperm cells are in the fallopian tubes when the egg is released—making it easier for fertilization to occur. Sperm can survive in the female reproductive tract for up to four or five days.

The best way to increase your chances of getting pregnant is to ensure that you're having sex at the right time in your cycle.

If you have regular cycles, you will ovulate around two weeks before your period. This means your fertile window will be seven days before your expected ovulation.

Tracking your cycle and your basal body temperature will give you the understanding of where your ovulation window occurs, which will allow the best chance of getting pregnant.

If you have irregular cycles, it can be a little more challenging to predict when you will ovulate and when your fertile window will be. This is why it is so essential to track your cycle using Clue, Kindara or even using a good old-fashioned pen and paper. Using these tools will enable you to see a trend of when you have your fertile window.

There are several techniques that you can use to predict your fertility and ovulation window.

- Ovulation predictor kit (not sure how reliable these are)
- Basal body temperature (temperature can rise by even half a degree, and this can be a sign you have ovulated)
- Cervical mucus changes
- Follicular monitoring

Please realise that if you are on contraception, this

prevents pregnancy from happening. So if you are looking to conceive, please check in with your doctor to guide you on how to come off contraception and the time frame that it may involve. Please see the Chapter on the Pill for more details on this.

Symptoms of pregnancy

You may notice some signs and symptoms before you even take a pregnancy test. Others will appear weeks later as your hormone levels change.

- Missed period
- Headache
- Spotting
- Weight gain
- Pregnancy-induced hypertension
- Heartburn
- Constipation
- Cramps
- Back pain
- Anaemia
- Depression
- Insomnia
- Breast changes
- Acne
- Vomiting
- Hip pain
- Diarrhoea
- Stress

If you think you may be pregnant, you shouldn't rely solely on these signs and symptoms for confirmation. Taking a home pregnancy test or seeing your doctor for lab testing can confirm a possible pregnancy. Many of these signs and symptoms can also be caused by other conditions like premenstrual syndrome (PMS). Learn more about the early symptoms of pregnancy — such as how soon they'll appear after you miss your period.

Pregnancy week by week

First Trimester – 0 to 12 weeks

Week 1	Week 6
Date of last period/missed period	The pregnancy test is positive
The placenta begins to develop	Eyes formed
Brain & Major organs form	Muscles develop
	Ear structure forms
	Foetus forms

Second Trimester – 12 to 25 weeks

Week 14	Week 21
Sex Identifiable	Vernix forming
Heartbeat audibles	The baby is growing in size
Scalp hair forming	

Third Trimester – 25 to 42 weeks

Week 28	Week 29
Foetus able to hiccup	Fat layers forming
	Organs mature
	Eye Split
	Hearing is more acute.

Week 34	Week 40-42
Kidneys Mature	(Estimated) Due Date
Lungs mature	Barbie protective tissues and hair disappear in preparation for birth
Weight increases by 200 grams weekly	

It is important to know that every pregnancy is different, but developments will most likely occur within this general time frame. Find out more about the changes you and your baby will undergo throughout the trimesters.

Your doctor or midwife will be able to talk you through the different stages at the various scans in a lot more detail.

The Pill and other hormonal birth control methods

Birth control pills, patches and the vaginal ring work by controlling the hormone levels in a woman's body. They're available by prescription. Other forms of hormonal birth control include the patch and the vaginal ring. They're also available by prescription, and their effectiveness rates are similar to those of the Pill.

Condoms

Condoms, diaphragms, and sponges are convenient and inexpensive forms of birth control that can be bought without a prescription. They're most effective when used correctly every time you have sexual intercourse.

Condoms are the only birth control method that both prevent pregnancy and protect against STDs. Discover the safest condoms on the market here.

Please check the chapter on the pill for more detail.

Nutrition for Pregnancy

A good diet is vital in life, but especially in preparation for pregnancy. Eating well before and during the pregnancy will help you and your baby start life with all the nutrients required to maintain all bodily functions and health during and after the delivery.

Now is not the time to diet. It is not recommended for overweight or obese women to start dieting when you fall pregnant as it can be harmful to the unborn baby.

If you are overweight, you can safely gain less than 0.5kg a week, as long as you are eating good food and having regular meals (breakfast, lunch and dinner). This means you have enough nourishment (calcium, iron, vitamins, protein and energy) for your baby's healthy development. If you do not eat enough wholesome food, you and your baby miss out.

During pregnancy, macronutrient intake needs to grow significantly. Macronutrients include carbohydrates, proteins, and fats.

For example, protein intake needs to increase from the recommended 0.36 grams per pound (0.8 grams per kg) of body weight for non-pregnant women to 0.5 grams per pound (1.1 grams per kg) of body weight for pregnant women. There are varying recommendations so please just aim for regular portions of protein where possible.

You'll want to be including protein in every meal and snack to meet your needs.

The requirement for micronutrients, including vitamins, minerals, and trace elements, increases even more than they need for macronutrients.

While some people can meet this growing demand through a well-planned, nutrient-dense eating plan, others can find it challenging.

You may need to take vitamin and mineral

supplements for various reasons, including:

- *Nutrient deficiencies*: Some people may need a supplement after a blood test reveals a deficiency in a vitamin or mineral. Correcting deficiencies is critical, as a shortage of nutrients like folate are linked to congenital disabilities.

- *Hyperemesis gravidarum:* This pregnancy complication is characterized by severe nausea and vomiting. It can lead to weight loss and nutrient deficiencies.

- *Dietary restrictions:* Women who follow specific diets, including vegans and those with food intolerances and allergies, may need to supplement with vitamins and minerals to prevent micronutrient deficiencies.

- *Smoking:* Although it's critical for mothers to avoid cigarettes during pregnancy, those who continue to smoke have an increased need for specific nutrients like vitamin C and folate.

- *Multiple pregnancies:* Women carrying more than one baby have higher micronutrient needs than women carrying one baby. Supplementing is often necessary to ensure optimal nutrition for both the mother and her babies.

- *Genetic mutations like MTHFR*: Methylenetetrahydrofolate reductase

(MTHFR) is a gene that converts folate into a form that the body can use. Pregnant women with this gene mutation may need to supplement with a specific form of folate to avoid complications.

- *Poor nutrition:* Women who undereat or choose foods low in nutrients may need to supplement with vitamins and minerals to avoid deficiencies.

In addition, experts like those at the American College of Obstetricians and Gynaecologists (ACOG) recommend that all pregnant people take a prenatal vitamin and folic acid supplement. This is advised to fill nutritional gaps and prevent developmental abnormalities at birth like spina bifida.

You can stay at a healthy weight by eating healthily and exercising. You will gain about 0.5 kg (1lb) a week during the second and third trimester. Currently, there are no evidence-based policy guidelines on recommended weight gain for women during pregnancy. Please check with your doctor regularly during the pregnancy.

Nutrition

Before I go any further it is important to note that eating for two is a myth. The energy requirement does not change during the 1st 6 months of pregnancy. During the last 3 months of pregnancy, energy requirements increase by approximately 200 kcals per day.

Supplements that are considered safe during pregnancy.

Just as with medications, your doctor should approve and supervise all micronutrient and herbal supplements to ensure that they're necessary and taken in safe amounts.

Unfortunately, there isn't much research regarding the use of herbal supplements by pregnant women, and much is unknown about how the supplements can affect you.

My advice is to keep your doctor in the know about any changes to your eating plan and supplements.

1. Prenatal vitamins

Prenatal vitamins are multivitamins that are specially formulated to meet the increased demand for micronutrients during pregnancy.

They're intended to be taken before conception and during pregnancy and breastfeeding.

Observational studies have shown that supplementing with prenatal vitamins reduces the risk of preterm birth and preeclampsia. Preeclampsia is a potentially dangerous complication characterized by high blood pressure and possibly protein in the urine.

While prenatal vitamins aren't meant to replace your healthy eating plan, they may help prevent nutritional gaps by providing extra micronutrients that are in high demand during pregnancy.

Since prenatal vitamins contain the vitamins and minerals you'll need, taking additional vitamin or mineral supplements may not be necessary unless suggested by your doctor.

Prenatal vitamins are often prescribed by doctors and are available over-the-counter.

2. Folate

Folate is a B vitamin that plays an integral role in DNA synthesis, red blood cell production, and foetal growth and development.

Folic acid is the synthetic form of folate found in many supplements. It gets converted into the active form of folate — L-methyl folate — in the body.

It's recommended to take at least 400-600 micrograms (mcg) of folate or folic acid per day to reduce the risk of neural tube defects and congenital abnormalities like cleft palate and heart defects.

Another reason to be conscious of is that many pregnancies are unplanned, and birth abnormalities due to a folate deficiency can occur very early in pregnancy, even before most women know they're pregnant.

In a review of five randomized studies including 6,105 women, supplementing with folic acid daily was associated with a reduced risk of neural tube defects. No adverse side effects were noted.

Although adequate folate can be obtained through diet, many women don't eat enough folate-rich foods, making supplementation necessary.

It may be wise for pregnant women, especially those with an MTHFR genetic mutation, to choose a supplement that contains L-methyl folate to ensure maximum uptake.

Please consult your doctor for the best advice.

3. Iron

The need for iron increases significantly during pregnancy as maternal blood volume increases by about 45 per cent.

Iron is critical for oxygen transport and the healthy growth and development of your baby and the placenta.

In the United States, the prevalence of iron deficiency in pregnant women is around 18 per cent, and 5 percent of these women have anaemia. This is a lot more common than many realise.

Anaemia during pregnancy has been associated with preterm delivery, maternal depression, and infant anaemia.

The recommended intake of 27 milligrams (mg) of iron per day can be met through most prenatal vitamins. However, if you have iron deficiency or anaemia, you'll need higher doses of iron, managed by your doctor.

If you aren't iron deficient, you shouldn't take more than the recommended intake of iron to avoid adverse side effects. These may include constipation, vomiting, and abnormally high haemoglobin levels.

4. Vitamin D

This fat-soluble vitamin is essential for immune function, bone health, and cell division.

Vitamin D deficiency during pregnancy has been linked to an increased risk of caesarean section, preeclampsia, preterm birth, and gestational diabetes.

The current recommended intake of vitamin D during pregnancy is 600 IU or 15 mcg per day. However, some experts suggest that vitamin D needs during pregnancy are much higher.

Check-in with your doctor regarding screening for vitamin D deficiency and proper supplementation.

Even if you are not pregnant, taking Vitamin D between the months of October to March can have major benefits for your overall wellbeing.

5. Magnesium

Magnesium is a mineral involved in hundreds of chemical reactions in your body. It plays a critical role in immune, muscle, and nerve function.

Deficiency in this mineral during pregnancy may increase the risk of chronic hypertension and premature labour.

Some studies suggest that supplementing with magnesium may reduce the risk of complications like foetal growth restriction and preterm birth.

6. Ginger

Ginger root is commonly used as a spice and herbal supplement.

In supplement form, you may have heard of it to treat nausea caused by motion sickness, pregnancy, or chemotherapy.

A review of four studies suggested that ginger is safe and effective for treating pregnancy-induced nausea and vomiting.

Nausea and vomiting are common during pregnancy, with up to 80 per cent of women experiencing them in the First Trimester of pregnancy.

Though ginger may help reduce this unpleasant pregnancy complication, more research is needed to identify the maximum safe dosage. Double-check with your doctor to see if you need it.

7. Fish oil

Fish oil contains docosahexaenoic acid (DHA) and eicosapentaenoic acid (EPA), two essential fatty acids important for a baby's brain development.

Supplementing with DHA and EPA in pregnancy might boost post-pregnancy brain development in your baby and decrease maternal depression, though research on this topic isn't conclusive.

Although observational studies have shown improved cognitive function in the children of women supplementing with fish oil during pregnancy, several controlled studies have failed to show a consistent benefit.

For example, one 2010 study involving 2,399 women found no difference in the cognitive function of infants whose mothers had supplemented with fish oil capsules containing 800 mg of DHA per day during pregnancy compared with infants whose mothers did not.

This study also found that supplementing with fish oil did not affect maternal depression.

However, the study did find that supplementing with fish oil protected against preterm delivery, and some evidence suggests that fish oil may benefit foetal eye development.

Maternal DHA levels are essential for proper foetal development, and supplementing is considered safe. The jury is still out on whether taking fish oil during pregnancy is necessary.

To get DHA and EPA through food, it's encouraged to consume two to three servings of low-mercury fish like salmon, sardines, or pollock per week.

8. Probiotics

Given increased general awareness of gut health, many parents-to-be turn to probiotics.

Probiotics are living microorganisms that are thought to benefit digestive health.

Many studies have shown that probiotics are safe to take during pregnancy, and no harmful side effects have been identified, aside from an extremely low risk of probiotic-induced infection.

Additionally, several studies have shown that supplementing with probiotics may reduce the risk of gestational diabetes, postpartum depression, and infant eczema and dermatitis.

Research on probiotic use in pregnancy is ongoing, and more about the role of probiotics in maternal and foetal health is sure to be discovered.

Please consult with your doctor before taking any probiotic.

9. Choline

Choline plays a vital role in a baby's brain development and helps to prevent abnormalities of the brain and spine.

The current recommended daily allowance of choline during pregnancy (450 mg per day) has been thought to be inadequate and that an intake closer to 930 mg per day is optimal instead.

Note that prenatal vitamins often don't contain choline. Your doctor may recommend a separate choline supplement.

Supplements to avoid during pregnancy

While supplementing with some micronutrients and herbs is safe for pregnant women, many of them should be avoided or avoided in high amounts.

Always check with your doctor before adding any additional supplements outside of any prenatal vitamins you may be taking.

1. Vitamin A

You'll often find vitamin A in your prenatal vitamins since it's so important. Although this vitamin is essential for foetal vision development and immune function, too much vitamin A can be harmful.

Given that vitamin A is fat-soluble, your body stores excess amounts in the liver.

This accumulation can have toxic effects on the body and lead to liver damage. It can even cause congenital disabilities.

For example, excessive amounts of vitamin A during pregnancy has been shown to cause congenital birth abnormalities.

Between prenatal vitamins and foods, you should get enough vitamin A, and additional supplementation outside of your prenatal vitamins is not advised.

2. Vitamin E

This fat-soluble vitamin plays many vital roles in the body and is involved in gene expression and immune function.

While vitamin E is essential for health, it's recommended that you don't supplement with it.

Extra supplementation with vitamin E has not been shown to improve outcomes for either mothers or babies. It may instead increase the risk of abdominal pain and premature rupture of the amniotic sack.

3. Black cohosh

A member of the buttercup family, black cohosh is a plant used for various purposes, including controlling hot flashes and menstrual cramps.

It's unsafe to take this herb during pregnancy, as it can cause uterine contractions, inducing preterm labour.

Black cohosh has also been found to cause liver damage in some people.

4. Goldenseal

Goldenseal is a plant used as a dietary supplement to treat respiratory infections and diarrhoea, although there's very little research on its effects and safety.

Goldenseal contains a substance called berberine, which has been shown to worsen jaundice in infants.

It can lead to a condition called kernicterus, a rare type of brain damage that can be fatal.

For these reasons, definitely avoid goldenseal.

5. Yohimbe

Yohimbe is a supplement made from the bark of a tree native to Africa.

It's used as an herbal remedy to treat a range of conditions from erectile dysfunction to obesity.

This herb should never be used during pregnancy, as it has been associated with dangerous side effects like high blood pressure, heart attacks, and seizures.

7. Other herbal supplements considered unsafe during pregnancy

It's best to avoid the following:

- Saw palmetto
- Dong Quai
- Tansy
- Red clover
- Angelica
- Yarrow
- Wormwood
- Blue cohosh
- Pennyroyal
- Ephedra
- Mugwort

What about if you are vegan?

If you are currently on a vegan diet, women can continue with this during the pregnancy but will have to plan out meals to get all the nutrients they need.

Combine two or more of the following foods to achieve a well-balanced mixture of amino acids:

- Pulses – beans, lentils and peas
- Grains – Bread, pasts, rice, oats, breakfast cereals, corn and rye
- Nuts and seeds
- Quorn and soya products

Foods to Avoid

Several foods should be avoided for various reasons.

- *Soft or Blue cheeses (Roquefort, Camembert etc.)* – The mould in the cheese can contain listeria, which can cause food poisoning and can be harmful to the unborn baby.
- *Liver/Liver products or other products containing Vitamin A* – Too much Vitamin A can be toxic to the baby.
- *Swordfish, Marlin or Shark* – These types of fish can have very high levels of mercury, which can be harmful to the baby.
- *Pate, including veg pate* – May contain listeria.
- *Raw or uncooked food* - including meat, fish, shellfish. Unpasteurized foods such as eggs, homemade ice cream, homemade mayo or homemade cheesecake – These foods can cause salmonella. Please make sure all foods are piping hot before consumption.

- *Oily fish (sardines, salmon, tuna etc.)* – No more than two portions per week as large amounts of mercury can be harmful to the baby.
- *Caffeine* – Too much caffeine increases the risk of miscarriage and low birth weight babies. Please aim for no more than 200mg per day.
- *Alcohol* – Can increase the risk of miscarriage and low birth babies. No more than 1 or 2 units of alcohol, once or twice per week, and don't get drunk.

Pregnant women don't need to avoid the following:

- Shellfish, including prawns
- Live or bio yoghurt, Probiotic drinks or yoghurts, Fromage frais, Creme fraiche, Soured cream.
- Spicy foods
- Mayonnaise, ice cream, salad dressing (As long as they don't contain raw egg)
- Honey
- Many types of cheese, including; Cheddar, parmesan, feta, ricotta, mascarpone, cream cheese, mozzarella, cottage cheese, processed cheese such as cheese spreads
- Peanuts
- Herbal Teas

Dealing with Morning Sickness/Nausea

As mentioned before 80% of pregnant women can be prone to nausea. Here are a few tools that I have seen help clients to have a smoother pregnancy:

- *Stay hydrated* - Ice cold water or fruit juice really helps
- *Keep snacking* - Most people find that morning sickness is exacerbated by hunger. So eat first thing in the morning (have some oat cakes by your bedside), and keep snacking on some of the following throughout the day.
- *Try not to worry about missing the nutrients in your diet* - Vegetables, meat, fish and eggs are often a no-go zone for anyone with morning sickness. Instead, stock up on loads of fruit, and if you really want to get your green in - Pop some kale/spinach into your fruit smoothie - You won't taste it, I promise.
- *Smoothies* are also a great way of getting protein in - Add in full fat Greek yoghurt, milk or protein powder. And lots of ice - The colder the better!
- While snacking on the bland beige foods, try to make them as nutritious as possible. Switch wheat crackers for oat cakes. Switch white pasta for spelt pasta. Switch white rice for brown rice. And instead of a white loaf of bread, whip up some homemade oat bread
- Ginger tea and Ginger Oatcakes are some of my pregnant clients' faves! Again, it just means you're getting more nutrients in comparison to Gingernut biscuits!
- *Vitamin B6* has been shown to be effective in helping morning sickness. Make sure there's

about 25-30mcg in your pregnancy. And make sure you have a pregnancy multi that doesn't repeat on you! Take it with a snack

These tips are for morning sickness, of course if you have severe hyperemesis gravidarum you may need to go chat with your consultant or midwife.

Weight Management after Pregnancy

A gradual weight loss (0.5-1kg per week) after pregnancy will not affect the ability to breastfeed or the quality or quantity of the milk produced.

Mothers should be encouraged to wait until their 6-8 postnatal check before embarking on any physical activity regime. However, if the pregnancy and labour were normal with no complications, walking, pelvic floor exercises, and gentle stretches can begin immediately.

Women should be encouraged to return to their pre-pregnancy weight but to expect this to happen gradually. Fad diets, quick fixes and crash diets are not recommended.

Please seek doctors' advice on this. A healthy diet and regular physical activity should be encouraged after birth.

Breastfeeding

Breastfeeding is encouraged, and exclusive breastfeeding for the first 6 months of life is recommended. Women should be encouraged to breastfeed. Breastfeeding will always be the mother's choice. Someone who I highly recommend to contact is Nicola O'Byrne (@nicola_lactationconsultant on Instagram).

The research concludes that exclusive breastfeeding for the first 5 months after birth requires an extra 625 kcal/day, so please ensure that you are fuelling your body during this time.

During breastfeeding, women are encouraged to eat a balanced and varied diet. During this phase, Breastfeeding women can now consume many of the foods they were unable to enjoy during pregnancy, such as; Soft cheeses, pate, rare meat etc. However, they should still limit oily fish to no more than twice per week and limit shark, swordfish and marlin to no more than once per week.

Aim to have regular drinks throughout the day, including water, milk, and a small amount of pure fruit juice are good options. Alcohol will pass through the breast milk to the baby and should ideally be avoided. If drinking alcohol, aim for no more than 1-2 units once or twice a week and ideally avoid alcohol for at least 2 hours before breastfeeding.

Caffeine can also pass to the baby when breastfeeding and may cause the baby to become unsettled, avoiding or limiting tea, coffee and other drinks containing caffeine.

Exercise

We all know at this stage that exercise is good for us. It can aid our sleep, improve mood, improve energy, decrease labour and quicker recovery and promote muscle tone, strength, and endurance.

Before undertaking the overall health of the woman should be reviewed before any exercise programme can be started. So please check with your doctor before doing anything.

Recommendation for Pregnant Clients:

If you have recently had a baby (first of all congratulations) and you are looking to get a coach/PT please make sure they are qualified to work with Pre and Post Natal women. If someone is not qualified, please stay away. All the coaches that work under my branding are qualified to help.

You must get signed off by a doctor to make sure everything is ok. Consider using resistance bands, medicine balls, suspension units, stability balls and BOSUs for training. It all depends on initial fitness levels. If you haven't been training before pregnancy during it may not be a fantastic idea to start.

Meditation and other relaxation techniques are hugely beneficial.

Resistance training

If you have been training before, you may have been used to pushing yourself hard in the gym. During pregnancy is not the time to do this. A training program should be designed for you and must have clearance from a medical professional.

The program itself:

- Maximum 2 exercises per body part and max 3 sets of each
- Increase rest to 2 mins
- Do not train to failure
- Chose a lightweight which can be performed for 15 reps and only do 8/10 reps
- Reduce bench-based exercises
- Reduce lunges or Squats (if you have been squatting with weight before, please continue)
- Machine-based exercises are safer
- Don't breathe hold
- Heart rate shouldn't go above 140 BPM (this varies on levels of fitness of the individual)
- Max 3 days per week (depending on starting fitness levels)
- 30 – 40 mins max depending on how you feel
- Swimming and cycling are excellent as there is no added weight

Recommendations for Post Natal Clients:

Please note that these are recommendations and may or may not apply to everyone.

0-3 weeks Post Natal:

- Should include walking, postnatal core and pelvic floor exercises

3-8 weeks Post Natal:

- Should consist of walking and swimming (once bleeding has stopped)
- Gyms programs – maintain posture, lightweights, no breath-holding
- Postnatal ab and pelvic floor exercises
- Low impact aerobics or a postnatal class
- Low-intensity water aerobics (once bleeding has stopped)

8-12 weeks Postnatal:

- Same as 3-8 weeks, but we can increase intensity or weight lifted. Progress postnatal core. Ab and pelvic floor exercises

12- 16 weeks Postnatal:

- Ab and pelvic floor muscle testing before return to higher impact exercise, running, sport and commencing regular ab exercise programmes. Note: Core strength should be close to normal at this stage.

16 weeks Postnatal

- Return to previous levels providing pelvic floor muscles and core control levels are back to normal. Group classes (Pre and Post -Natal) are a great option for mothers and expectant mums as they provide considerable physical, emotional and social benefits.

Conclusion

Most healthy couples will conceive within a year of actively trying to get pregnant. If you don't get pregnant within a year and are under age 35, you should see your doctor for a fertility evaluation.

If you're over 35, you should only wait six months before seeing a doctor.

Couples should also see a fertility specialist if they have a history of multiple miscarriages or know that they have a genetic or medical condition that might affect their fertility.

It can be challenging when pregnancy doesn't happen right away, but try to be patient. This is normal. It doesn't mean that it'll never happen to you.

If you are coming off the pill and had a regular cycle before from research it shows that there is no negative effect on subsequent fertility. This research was carried out in a 2018 study, which looked at 14,884 women. The study showed that 83.1% women fell pregnant within 12-15 months after discontinuing the pill.

If you have conditions like PCOS, Endometriosis or have issues with cycle regularity please talk to your doctor for your options.

Try to keep up the baby-making fun, be adventurous, and stay relaxed.

Doing these things can help you increase your chances of getting that positive result you've been waiting for.

Achieving a healthy weight before conception should be encouraged for positive health outcomes for both the mother and the baby. Being overweight or obese before or during pregnancy can lead to health complications for both mother and baby.

Pregnant and breastfeeding women should be encouraged to eat a balanced, varied diet and participate in regular physical activity appropriate to their fitness and lifestyle.

Some food and drinks should be limited or avoided during pregnancy to protect the health of the mother and her unborn child.

The nutrition a mother receives before she becomes pregnant, during gestation and beyond, will impact her health and that of her unborn child.

Evidence shows that exercise is safer for both mother and fetus during pregnancy in most cases, and women should therefore be encouraged to initiate and continue to train for added health benefits.

Please check in with medical professionals along the way.

Chapter 8 - Perimenopause and Menopause

Lara Briden sums up the next chapter of a woman's life brilliantly when she called it the 2nd puberty. Puberty as we all know is a time when your body changes, we feel a little off mentally and sometimes insecurities can be heightened. This is very similar to what perimenopause and menopause bring.

Although the life stage of Menopause is well known, there are actually different stages within menopause that are important to recognize and understand. Menopause itself officially occurs when you stop menstruating for 12 months.

Perimenopause, on the other hand, means "around menopause." It's also known as the menopause transitional phase and is called such because it happens before menopause.

Although they're both part of the same overall life transition, menopause and perimenopause have different symptoms and treatment options.

So, let's look into the differences in symptoms.

Perimenopause

What are the signs of perimenopause?

You're in your 40s, you wake up in a sweat at night, and your periods are erratic and often accompanied by heavy bleeding: Chances are, you're going through perimenopause.
Many women experience an array of symptoms as their hormones shift during the months or years leading up to menopause — that is, the natural end

of menstruation. Menopause is a point in time, but perimenopause (peri, Greek for "around" or "near" + menopause) is an extended transitional state.

What is perimenopause?

Perimenopause has been variously defined, but experts generally agree that it begins with irregular menstrual cycles — courtesy of declining ovarian function — and ends a year after the last menstrual period.

Perimenopause varies greatly from one woman to the next. This is why it is essential that you are in tune with your body and your cycles from early on. This will allow you to spot any irregularities that may occur. The average duration is three to four years, although it can last just a few months or extend as long as a decade.

Some women feel buffeted by hot flashes and wiped out by heavy periods; many have no bothersome symptoms. Periods may end more or less abruptly for some, while others may menstruate erratically for years. Fortunately, as knowledge about reproductive aging has grown, so have the options for treating some of its more distressing features.

Perimenopause and Estrogen

During your peak reproductive years, the amount of estrogen in circulation rises and falls fairly predictably throughout the menstrual cycle. Estrogen levels are largely controlled by two hormones, follicle-stimulating hormone (FSH) and luteinizing hormone (LH). FSH stimulates the follicles — the fluid-filled sacs in the ovaries that contain the eggs — to produce estrogen.

When estrogen reaches a certain level, the brain signals the pituitary to turn off the FSH and produce a surge of LH. This in turn stimulates the ovary to release the egg from its follicle (ovulation). The leftover follicle produces progesterone, in addition to estrogen, in preparation for pregnancy. As these hormone levels rise, the levels of FSH and LH drop. If pregnancy doesn't occur, progesterone falls, menstruation takes place, and the cycle begins again.

As peri menopause is kicking in estrogen does not decrease in a gradual decline it's more erratic than that. I compare it to the stock market, the estrogen could be high at some points and lower at others.

It is essential that we are aware the sequence of events with perimenopause:

1. Lower estrogen
2. High and fluctuating estrogen
3. Lower estrogen
4. Possible insulin resistance

On average, the entire natural perimenopause transition takes about 7 years.

In fact, according to the Cleveland Clinic, hormonal changes are seen 8 to 10 years ahead of menopause. This happens during your 30s or 40s even before the onset of perimenopause.

During the final stages of perimenopause, your body will produce less and less estrogen. Despite the sharp drop in estrogen, it's still possible to get pregnant. Perimenopause can last for as little as a few months and as long as 4 years.

It is important to be aware that there is such a thing as early onset menopause. If you reach menopause before the age of 45 or undergo menopause that is surgically or medically induced, you will not experience many of these symptoms but you will be moved directly to a lower estrogen state.

If you have had a procedure called a hysterectomy (removal of the uterus). But retain your ovaries and you will experience many of the symptoms.

Menopause officially kicks in when the ovaries produce so little estrogen that eggs are no longer released. This also causes your period to stop.

Your doctor will diagnose menopause once you haven't had a period for a full year.

You may enter menopause earlier than normal if you:

- have a family history of early menopause
- are a smoker
- have had a hysterectomy or oophorectomy
- have undergone cancer treatments
- Symptoms of perimenopause and menopause

When it comes to menopause, most people think about the symptoms more than anything else. These can include those infamous hot flashes, but there are many other changes you might experience during this transition.

Symptoms of perimenopause may include:

- irregular periods
- periods that are heavier or lighter than normal
- worse premenstrual syndrome (PMS) before periods
- breast tenderness
- weight gain
- hair changes
- heart palpitations
- headaches
- loss of sex drive
- concentration difficulties
- forgetfulness
- muscle aches
- urinary tract infections (UTIs)
- fertility issues in women who are trying to conceive

Menopause symptoms

As estrogen levels drop, you might start experiencing symptoms of menopause. Some of these can occur while you're still at the perimenopause stage.

- night sweats
- hot flashes
- depression

- anxiety or irritability
- mood swings
- insomnia
- fatigue
- dry skin
- vaginal dryness
- frequent urination
- cholesterol

In some studies Perimenopause and menopause can also increase cholesterol levels. This is one reason why women in post menopause are at an even higher risk for heart disease. Please continue to have your cholesterol levels measured at least once a year.

Treatments for symptoms

Hot flashes

Hot flashes are one of the most frequent symptoms of menopause. Up to 75% of women experience them. It is a brief sensation of heat. Hot flashes aren't the same for everyone and there's no definitive reason that they happen. Aside from the heat, hot flashes can also come with:

- A red, flushed face.
- Sweating.
- A chilled feeling after the heat.

Hot flashes not only feel different for each woman — they also can last for various amounts of time. Some women only have hot flashes for a short period of time during menopause. Others can have some kind of hot flash for the rest of their life. Typically, hot flashes are less severe as time goes on.

If you are suffering with flashes there are steps that you can take to manage certain menopausal symptoms:

- Turn down your thermostat.
- Wear light layers of clothing.
- Have a fan handy to mitigate hot flashes and night sweats.

Here are a few other methods you can try to relieve symptoms:

- Pay attention to your diet and avoid large meals.
- Quit smoking, if you smoke.
- Only drink alcohol in moderation.
- Limit caffeine to small quantities and only have it in the morning.

What triggers a hot flash?

There are quite a few normal things in your daily life that could set off a hot flash. Some things to look out for include:

- Caffeine
- Smoking
- Spicy foods
- Alcohol
- Tight clothing
- Stress and anxiety

- Heat, including hot weather, can also trigger a hot flash. Be careful when working out in hot weather — this could cause a hot flash.

If you are experiencing any of the symptoms below then it is essential that you go and talk to your doctor

Other symptoms that may occur include:

- spotting after your period
- blood clots during your period
- bleeding after sex
- periods that are much longer or much shorter than normal

Some possible explanations are hormonal imbalances or fibroids, both of which are treatable. However, you also want to rule out the possibility of cancer.

You should also call your doctor if the symptoms of either perimenopause or menopause become severe enough to interfere with your daily life.

Treatments for perimenopause and menopause

There are both prescription and over-the-counter (OTC) treatments available for perimenopause and menopause.

Estrogen

Estrogen (hormone) therapy works by normalizing

estrogen levels so sudden hormonal spikes and drops don't cause uncomfortable symptoms. Some forms of estrogen may even help reduce the risk of osteoporosis.

Estrogen is available over the counter or by prescription.

Estrogen is usually combined with progestin and comes in many forms, including:

- oral pills
- creams
- gels
- skin patches

Other menopause medications are more targeted. For example:

- Prescription vaginal creams can alleviate dryness as well as pain from intercourse.
- Antidepressants can help with mood swings.
- The seizure medication gabapentin (Neurontin) can be an option for hot flashes.

Home remedies for perimenopause and menopause

There are also methods you can use to alleviate your symptoms at home.

The importance of regular Exercise
Exercise can help improve your mood, weight gain issues, and even (ironically) your hot flashes. Plan to include some form of physical activity in your daily routine.

Every woman experience menopause differently. For some, the symptoms are mild and pass quickly. For others, it's an explosion of hot flashes and mood swings.

The good news is you can adopt lifestyle changes to help cope with the changes occurring in your body.

Regular exercise is also an excellent way to stave off weight gain and loss of muscle mass, which are two frequent symptoms of menopause.

Most healthy women should aim for at least 150 minutes of moderate aerobic activity, or 75 minutes of vigorous aerobic activity a week, according to the Centres for Disease Control and Prevention (CDC).

What's the best form of exercise?

Cardio

Aerobic activity that makes use of your large muscle groups while keeping up your heart rate is a good thing. Your options for cardio are limitless. Almost any activity counts, for example:

- walking
- jogging
- biking
- Swimming

The CDC recommends that beginners start with 10

minutes of light activity, slowly boosting exercise intensity as it becomes easier. The likes of swimming and biking are great if you have issues with joints as they are less taxing on the body.

Strength training

Because osteoporosis risk skyrockets following menopause (estrogen is needed to help lay down bone), strength training is especially vital. Strength training exercises will help to build bone and muscle strength and improve overall body composition over time.

HIIT Training

HIIT stands for high intensity interval training (HIIT) is alternating short periods of really hard anaerobic work (think 85-95% of your maximum heart rate) followed by less intense recovery (around 70% - not all the way down). The maximum session duration is usually about 30 minutes - and you should feel pretty exhausted.

High intensity work can help to increase blood glucose control, boost your body's ability to downgrade inflammation, and improve your brain cognition and memory. Now this does not mean you have to jump around a living room over and over again. This just means that throwing in some higher intensity cardio could aid over all fitness and help you on your journey. If you are someone who suffers with issues with joints etc you may be able to do this style of exercise on a stationary bike or other similar forms of equipment.

Yoga and meditation

As no two women experience menopause in the same way, your unique symptoms will tailor your approach to relief. Practice a relaxation technique that works for you — whether it's deep breathing, yoga, or meditation.

Supported and restorative yoga poses may offer some relief. They can also help alleviate symptoms such as:

- hot flashes
- irritability
- Fatigue

Dancing

Exercise shouldn't be entirely hard work. Packing a session into your routine can be fun and good for your body and can be a great way of meeting new people.
If running on a treadmill isn't your thing, consider a dance class.

Be realistic

Set goals to avoid frustration. Make sure your goals are:

- realistic
- attainable
- specific

Don't simply declare, "I'm going to exercise more." Tell yourself, for example:

- "I'll walk for 30 minutes at lunch three days a week."
- "I'll take a group cycling class."
- "I'll play tennis with a friend once a week."

Recruit a friend or your spouse as a workout buddy to help keep you motivated and accountable.

Exercise is amazing for many things and as a woman's risk for numerous medical conditions, including breast cancer, type 2 diabetes, and heart disease rises during and after menopause. Working out regularly and maintaining a healthy weight can help offset these risks.

You can train at home with some home equipment (kettlebell and or dumbbells) or train in the gym, choosing from weight machines or free weights. The added benefit of lifting weights is that it will help you give you that toned look (toned means building muscle). Start off slow and try not to do what a lot of people do after Christmas which is go hell for leather and then never return again. If you are new to training, hire a coach.

Nutrition

Nutrition as we all know plays a massive role no matter what stage of life you are at.

There is evidence that certain foods may help relieve some symptoms of menopause, such as hot flashes, poor sleep and low bone density.

Dairy Products

The decline in estrogen levels during menopause can increase women's risk of fractures.

Dairy products, such as milk, yogurt and cheese, contain calcium, phosphorus, potassium, magnesium and vitamins D and K — all of which are essential for bone health.

In a study in nearly 750 postmenopausal women, those who ate more dairy and animal protein had significantly higher bone density than those who ate less.
Dairy may also help improve sleep. A review study found that foods high in the amino acid glycine — found in milk and cheese, for example — promoted deeper sleep-in menopausal women.

Furthermore, some evidence links dairy consumption to a decreased risk of premature menopause, which occurs before the age of 45.
In one study, women with the highest intake of vitamin D and calcium — which cheese and fortified milk are rich in — had a 17% reduced risk of early menopause.

Healthy Fats

Healthy fats, such as omega-3 fatty acids, may

benefit women going through menopause.

Still, it may be worth testing if increasing your omega-3 intake improves your menopause-related symptoms. See more details in the supplementation section.

Foods's highest in omega-3 fatty acids include fatty fish, such as mackerel, salmon and anchovies, and seeds like flax seeds, chia seeds and hemp seeds.

Whole Grains

Whole grains are high in nutrients, including fibre and B vitamins, such as thiamine, niacin, riboflavin and pantothenic acid.

A diet high in whole grains has been linked to a reduced risk of heart disease, cancer and premature death.

In a review, researchers found that people who ate three or more servings of whole grains per day had a 20–30% lower risk of developing heart disease and diabetes, compared to people who ate mostly refined carbs.

A study in over 11,000 postmenopausal women noted that eating 4.7 grams of whole-grain fibre per 2,000 calories per day reduced the risk of early death by 17%, compared to eating only 1.3 grams of whole-grain fibre per 2,000 calories.

Whole-grain foods include brown rice, whole-wheat bread, barley, quinoa, and rye. Look for "whole grain" listed as the first ingredient on the label when evaluating which packaged foods contain primarily whole grains. This is not to say to avoid white starchy carbohydrates. Wholegrain has shown evidence that they may be more beneficial for you over all.

PS carbs will not make you fat!

Fruits and Vegetables

Fruits and vegetables are packed with vitamins and minerals, fibre and antioxidants. For this reason, American dietary guidelines recommend filling half your plate with fruits and vegetables.

In a one-year intervention study in over 17,000 menopausal women, those eating more vegetables, fruit, fibre and soy experienced a 19% reduction in hot flashes compared to the control group. The reduction was attributed to the healthier diet and weight loss.

Cruciferous vegetables may be especially helpful for postmenopausal women. In one study, eating broccoli decreased levels of a type of estrogen linked to breast cancer, while increasing levels of an estrogen type that protects against breast cancer.

Dark berries may also benefit women going through menopause. In an eight-week study in 60 menopausal women, 25 grams a day of freeze-dried strawberry powder lowered blood pressure compared to a control group. However, more research is needed.

In another eight-week study in 91 middle-aged women, those who took 200 mg of grape seed extract supplements daily experienced fewer hot flashes, better sleep and lower rates of depression, compared to a control group.

Phytoestrogen-Containing Foods

Phytoestrogens are compounds in foods that act as weak estrogens in your body.

While there has been some controversy on including these in the diet, the most recent research suggests they may benefit health — especially for women going through menopause.

Foods that naturally contain phytoestrogens include soybeans, chickpeas, peanuts, flax seeds, barley, grapes, berries, plums, green and black tea and many more.

In a review of 21 studies on soy, postmenopausal women who took soy isoflavone supplements for at least four weeks had 14% higher estradiol (estrogen) levels compared to those who took a placebo. However, the results were not significant.

In another review of 15 studies ranging from 3 to 12 months, phytoestrogens including soy, isoflavone supplements and red clover were found to lower incidences of hot flashes compared to control groups, with no serious side effects.

Quality Protein

The decline in estrogen from menopause is linked to

decreased muscle mass and bone strength.

For this reason, women going through menopause should eat more protein. Aiming for regular portions of protein per day (each meal ideally) is a great place to start.

In a large study in adults over 50, eating dairy protein was linked to an 8% lower risk of hip fracture, while eating plant protein was linked to a 12% reduction.

Foods's high in protein include eggs, meat, fish, legumes and dairy products. Additionally, you can add protein powders to smoothies or baked goods.

Incorporating dairy products, healthy fats, whole grains, fruits, vegetables, foods high in phytoestrogens and quality sources of protein into your diet may help relieve some menopause symptoms.

Foods to watch out for

Reducing certain foods may help reduce some of the symptoms linked to menopause, such as hot flashes, weight gain and poor sleep.

Reducing Carbs

Reducing carbs does not mean take out or restrict. That is not my philosophy. Think of it like when you are approaching a set of traffic lights you reduce your speed you don't just jam down the breaks. Well, you're not meant to!

It is important to note that some women depending on genetic factors, age etc may struggle to break down certain carbs and be insulin resistant. This does not mean to stay off carbs, this means that it is normally danger in the dose and wholegrain options more often than not may help you more.

Although it may take some time to adjust to the processes taking place in your body, try to do your best to accept these changes that will inevitably happen with age.

Alcohol and Caffeine

Studies have shown that caffeine and alcohol can trigger hot flashes in women going through menopause.

In one study in 196 menopausal women, caffeine and alcohol intake increased the severity of hot flashes but not their frequency.

On the other hand, another study associated caffeine intake with a lower incidence of hot flashes.

Therefore, it may be worth testing whether eliminating caffeine affects your hot flashes. Another factor to consider is that caffeine and alcohol are known sleep disruptors and that many women goings through menopause have trouble sleeping. So, if this is the case for you, consider avoiding caffeine or alcohol near bedtime.

Spicy Foods

Avoiding spicy foods is a common recommendation for women going through menopause. However, evidence to support this is limited.

One study in 896 women going through menopause in Spain and South America examined the association between lifestyle factors and incidences of hot flashes and associated spicy food intake with an increase in hot flashes.

Another study in 717 perimenopausal women in India associated hot flashes with spicy food intake and anxiety levels. Researchers concluded that hot flashes were worse for women with overall poorer health.

As your reaction to spicy foods may be individual, use your best judgment when it comes to including spicy foods in your diet and avoid them if they seem to worsen your symptoms.

High-Salt Foods

High salt intake has been linked to lower bone density in postmenopausal women.

In a study in over 9,500 postmenopausal women, sodium intake of more than 2 grams per day was linked to a 28% higher risk of low bone mineral density.

Additionally, after menopause, the decline in estrogen increases your risk of developing high blood pressure. Reducing your sodium intake may help lower this risk.

Furthermore, in a randomized study in 95 postmenopausal women, those who followed a moderate-sodium diet experienced better overall mood, compared to women who followed a generally healthy diet with no salt restriction. Reducing processed carbs, alcohol, caffeine, spicy foods and foods high in salt may improve symptoms of menopause.

Menopause is linked to changes in metabolism, reduced bone density and increased risk of heart disease.

Additionally, many women going through menopause experience unpleasant symptoms, such as hot flashes and poor sleep.

A whole-foods diet high in fruits, vegetables, whole grains, high-quality protein and dairy products may reduce menopause symptoms. Phytoestrogens and healthy fats, such as omega-3 fatty acids from fish, may also help.

You may want to reduce added sugars, processed carbs, alcohol, caffeine and high-sodium or spicy foods as well.

These simple changes to your diet may make this important transition in your life easier.
Supplements

There is growing interest in botanical and other nutritional supplements to treat menopausal symptoms. Some of these supplements include:

Magnesium

Magnesium is an important mineral in the human body. It influences mood regulation, sleep, supports healthy bones and hormone levels, and is involved in hundreds of biochemical reactions throughout your body.

What's more, as women reach older adulthood and experience menopause, magnesium becomes particularly important for good health and may even help reduce menopause symptoms.

Most menopausal women have inadequate magnesium levels, putting them at greater risk of poor health. However, magnesium can be consumed through many foods, such as dark chocolate, beans, lentils, nuts, seeds, leafy greens, and whole grains.

You can also easily find magnesium supplements over the counter or online. For most people, they're considered safe for use, but be sure to consult your healthcare provider first.

Normally a dosage of 100mg-420mg per day is a safe place to start but some may need more. This is the gold standard supplement for menopause symptoms.

Omega-3 fatty acids

A review study in 483 menopausal women concluded that omega-3 supplements decreased the frequency of hot flashes and the severity of night sweats.

However, in another review of 8 studies on omega-3 and menopausal symptoms, only a few studies supported the beneficial effect of the fatty acid on hot flashes. Therefore, the results were inconclusive.
Still, it may be worth testing if increasing your omega-3 intake improves your menopause-related symptoms.

Foods's highest in omega-3 fatty acids include fatty fish, such as mackerel, salmon and anchovies, and seeds like flax seeds, chia seeds and hemp seeds. If you find that you struggle to get enough of these foods, supplementation can be beneficial.

Vitamin D & Calcium

Daily combined doses of 1,000 to 1,200 grams of calcium and 400 to 800 IU of vitamin D have been found to reduce overall fracture risk by 6% and hip fracture risk by 16%.

Creatine

Creatine is a substance that's found naturally in your muscles. It has been shown to help with exercise recovery, as well as improve strength, power, muscle mass, and anaerobic exercise capacity.

In women specifically, creatine supplements have been linked to improvements in strength, exercise performance, and muscle mass, both pre- and postmenopause.

Furthermore, early research suggests that taking creatine supplements may have benefits for women outside of the gym, including helping reduce mental fatigue and manage depression.

Aiming for 3-5g per day is where to start. Please make sure to increase your water intake alongside this.

Vitex agnus-castus (chasteberry)

Vitex agnus-castus is a popular herbal supplement used to treat a variety of health problems. For instance, Vitex agnus-castus is used to treat:

- PMS
- symptoms of menopause
- infertility issues
- other conditions affecting a woman's reproductive system

The hormone-balancing effects of Vitex agnus-castus may also help relieve symptoms of menopause.

In one study, vitex oils were given to 23 women in menopause. Women reported improved menopause symptoms, including better mood and sleep. Some even regained their period.
In a follow-up study 52 additional pre- and postmenopausal women were given a vitex cream. Of the study participants, 33 percent experienced major improvements, and another 36 percent

reported moderate improvements in symptoms, including night sweats and hot flashes.

However, not all studies have observed benefits. One recent and larger double-blind, randomized, controlled trial — the gold standard in research — gave women a placebo or a daily tablet containing a combination of vitex and St. John's wort.

After 16 weeks, the vitex supplement was no more effective than the placebo at reducing hot flashes, depression or any other menopausal symptoms.

Keep in mind that in many studies reporting benefits, women were provided with supplements that mixed Vitex agnus-castus with other herbs. Therefore, it's difficult to isolate the effects of vitex alone. The research is promising on this but more is needed to provide a definitive answer and needs to be further backed up by science.

Other supplements that research has looked into include Creatine, dehydroepiandrosterone (DHEA), evening primrose oil, soy isoflavones and St. John's wort.

The effectiveness of these supplements is variable. For example, some women find relief from hot flashes by supplementing soy isoflavones, but some women experience no benefits. This may be because certain gut bacteria metabolize soy isoflavones into equol, a compound that exerts estrogenic effects. Women who don't benefit from supplementing soy isoflavones may be equol nonproducers, and they can take an equol supplement instead to see if this helps reduce their symptoms.

Black cohosh

Black Cohosh is a herb native to North America that has traditionally been used for cognitive and inflammatory conditions, but has grown in popularity due to it's ability to treat vasomotor symptoms of menopause; primarily hot flashes and night sweats.

If using an isopropanolic extract (usually sold under the brand name of Remifemin), 20-40mg daily is used in doses of 20mg; taking 20mg results in a once daily dosing, whereas taking 40mg is twice daily dosing of the 20mg. This dosage (20-40mg) confers 1-2mg of triterpenoid glycosides.

If using an aqueous:ethanolic extract of black cohosh root (i.e. not Remifemin) then doses range from 64-128mg daily which are usually taken in two divided doses. This contributed about the same amount of triterpenoid glycosides.

It is not known whether or not black cohosh needs to be taken with food, although it is sometimes recommended to do so out of prudence.

Red clover

Red Clover Extract (RCE) refers to any extract that is taken from the red clover plant, known botanically as trifolium pratense which is a good natural source of isoflavone molecules. There are a few brand name products of RCE (Promensil, Menoflavon, etc.)

Supplementation of Red Clover Extract tends to be 40mg of total isoflavones taken once a day, or two doses totalling 80mg a day. This can be reached through supplementing pure isoflavones (in which case the range is 40-80mg), supplementing brand name products such as Promensil, which confer 40mg isoflavones per 500mg capsule (so, around 8% isoflavones by weight) or approximately 5 grams of the whole plant without any particular extraction techniques.

When looking at research on RCE and menopausal symptoms, there are indeed benefits in isolated studies relative to placebo but there are also many failures indicating that supplementation is pretty unreliable in benefitting symptoms; this may be in part due to differences in absorption or simply due to potential industry bias (since many studies using the brand name products are partially funded by the producers of the products, and the independent studies tend to be more likely to report no significant benefit). There may be a minor reduction in anxiety however, which would be a perceived benefit and needs to be further evaluated. It should also be noted that most studies do report great benefit with supplementation, but the placebo effect per se is very prominent in studies on menopausal symptoms. More research is needed on RCE before we can make a definitive decision on it.
Certain vitamin and mineral supplementation may also be warranted during perimenopause and menopause. For example, declining reproductive hormones are associated with decreased bone

mineral density. In late perimenopause, bone loss accelerates, and menstrual cycles become more irregular. Daily combined doses of 1,000 to 1,200 grams of calcium and 400 to 800 IU of vitamin D have been found to reduce overall fracture risk by 6% and hip fracture risk by 16%.

My go for supplements alongside ensuring adequate protein are creatine and omegas.

Why do some women gain weight around menopause?

Weight gain at menopause is very common.

There are many factors at play, including:

- hormones
- aging
- lifestyle
- Genetics

However, the process of menopause is highly individual. It varies from woman to woman.

Before we go any further, we need a quick recap on the female reproductive life cycle
There are four periods of hormonal changes that occur during a woman's life.

These include:
- premenopause
- perimenopause
- menopause
- post menopause

1. Premenopause

Premenopause is the term for a woman's reproductive life while she's fertile. It begins at puberty, starting with the first menstrual period and ending with the last.

This phase lasts for approximately 30-40 years.

2. Perimenopause

Perimenopause literally means "around menopause." During this time, estrogen levels become erratic and progesterone levels decline.

A woman may start perimenopause anytime between her mid-30s and early 50s, but this transition typically occurs in her 40s and lasts 4–11 years.

Symptoms of perimenopause include:

- hot flashes and heat intolerance
- sleep disturbances
- menstrual cycle changes
- headaches
- mood changes, such as irritability
- depression
- anxiety
- weight gain

3. Menopause

Menopause officially occurs once a woman hasn't

had a menstrual period for 12 months. The average age of menopause is 51 years.

Up until then, she's considered perimenopausal.

Many women experience their worst symptoms during perimenopause, but others find that their symptoms intensify in the first year or two after menopause.

4. Post menopause

Post menopause begins immediately after a woman has gone 12 months without a period. The terms menopause and post menopause are often used interchangeably.

However, there are some hormonal and physical changes that may continue to occur after menopause.
A woman goes through hormonal changes throughout her lifetime that may produce symptoms, including changes in body weight.

Do changes in hormones affect metabolism?

During perimenopause, progesterone levels decline slowly and steadily, while estrogen levels fluctuate greatly from day to day and even within the same day.

In the early part of perimenopause, the ovaries often produce extremely high amounts of estrogen. This is due to impaired feedback signals between the ovaries, hypothalamus, and pituitary gland.

Later in perimenopause, when menstrual cycles become more irregular, the ovaries produce very little estrogen. They produce even less during menopause.

Some studies suggest that high estrogen levels may promote fat gain. This is because high estrogen levels are associated with weight gain and higher body fat during the reproductive years.

From puberty until perimenopause, women tend to store fat in their hips and thighs as subcutaneous fat. Although it can be hard to lose, this type of fat doesn't increase disease risk very much.

However, during menopause, low estrogen levels and higher testosterone levels promote fat storage in the belly area as visceral fat, which is linked to insulin resistance, type 2 diabetes, heart disease, and other health problems. This is why some women may see a shift of where they hold their fat to predominantly their stomach areas.

This is alongside eating in a consistent caloric surplus and reduced output through exercise.

Changes in hormone levels during the menopausal transition may lead to fat gain and an increased risk of several diseases. This could also be down to a decrease in metabolism, a decrease in exercise and an increase in calorie consumption. Once again calories in v calories out are king when it comes to gaining weight.

What weight changes during perimenopause?

It's estimated that women gain about 2–5 pounds (1–2 kgs) during the perimenopausal transition.

However, some gain more weight. This appears to be particularly true for women who are already overweight or have obesity.

Weight gain may also occur as part of aging, regardless of hormone changes.

Researchers looked at weight and hormone changes in women ages 42–50 over a 3-year period.

There was no difference in average weight gain between those who continued to have normal cycles and those who entered menopause.

The Study of Women's Health Across the Nation (SWAN) is a large observational study that has followed middle-aged women throughout perimenopause.

During the study, women gained belly fat and lost muscle mass.

Another factor contributing to weight gain in perimenopause may be the increased appetite and calorie intake that occurs in response to hormonal changes.

In one study, levels of the "hunger hormone,"

ghrelin, were found to be significantly higher among perimenopausal women, compared to premenopausal and postmenopausal women.

The low estrogen levels in the late stages of menopause may also impair the function of leptin and neuropeptide Y, hormones that control fullness and appetite.

Therefore, women in the late stages of perimenopause who have low estrogen levels may be driven to eat more calories.

Progesterone's effects on weight during the menopausal transition haven't been studied as much.

However, some researchers believe the combination of low estrogen and progesterone could further increase the risk of obesity.

Weight changes during and after menopause

Hormonal changes and weight gain may continue to occur as women leave perimenopause and enter menopause.

One predictor of weight gain may be the age at which menopause occurs.

A study of over 1,900 women found that those who entered menopause earlier than the average age of 51 had less body fat.

Additionally, there are several other factors that may contribute to weight gain after menopause.

Postmenopausal women are generally less active than when they were younger, which reduces energy expenditure and leads to a loss of muscle mass.

Menopausal women also frequently have higher fasting insulin levels and insulin resistance, which drive weight gain and increase heart disease risk.

Although its use is controversial, hormone replacement therapy has shown effectiveness in reducing belly fat and improving insulin sensitivity during and after menopause.

Keep in mind that the averages found in studies do not apply to all women. This varies between individuals.

Fat gain tends to occur during menopause as well. However, it's unclear if this is caused by an estrogen deficit or the aging process.

How to prevent weight gain around menopause
Here are a few things you can do to prevent weight gain around menopause:

- *Eat a balanced diet:* The rule of calories in vs calories out still plays a major factor.
- *Reduce carbs:* This doesn't mean restrict or take out means reduce the amount to see if you notice a difference in the management of insulin, as managing insulin may become a

factor. The total amount of calories will still be the biggest factor when gaining weight.
- *Add fibre:* Eat a high-fibre diet that includes flaxseeds, which may improve insulin sensitivity.
- *Work out:* Engage in strength training to improve body composition, increase strength, and build and maintain lean muscle.
- *Rest and relax:* Try to relax before bed and get enough sleep to keep your hormones and appetite well-managed.

If you follow these steps, it is possible to lose weight during this time.

Although weight gain is very common during menopause, there are steps you can take to prevent or reverse it.

Managing Sleep and Menopause

The hot flashes, night sweats, and anxiety experienced by many women with menopause are bad enough on their own, but when they start affecting your sleep, they can feel even worse. In a frustrating cycle, the stress and tiredness caused by another restless night can sometimes just make the symptoms, and your sleep problems, worse.

Many don't realise that if you don't get enough sleep (aiming for 7-9 hours is a decent amount) that affects our hunger and fullness hormones. It actually increases your hunger hormones and reduces the intensity of our fullness hormone. What generally happens then is that the brain will kick in and look for the quickest hit of energy, which invariably brings in foods like Carbs, Fats, sugar and processed foods.

There is nothing wrong with these foods (as a food cannot be good or bad) but these foods will not fill you. They will raise your blood sugar levels up and crash back down very quickly so you will be hungry quite quickly after and this cycle will be repeated.

Lifestyle changes can help you reduce the frequency of your hot flashes or make it easier to sleep through them. In some cases, your doctor may also prescribe hormone replacement therapy (HRT) or other treatments (look at the section on HRT for more information on this).

What's causing your sleep problems during menopause?

We just need a quick recap to what's going on as you near menopause, your ovaries stop producing the hormones estrogen and progesterone. The decrease in these hormones can cause hot flashes and night sweats. As your body's temperature begins to rise during sleep, you may wake up. By the time your hot flash has passed, you may have been awake for several uncomfortable minutes. Many women find it hard to fall back asleep afterward.

In addition to hot flashes and sweating, you may experience sleep problems as a result of depression, anxiety, or mood disorders during perimenopause or menopause. If you're facing extra emotional stress, the mental toll may prevent you from sleeping. If your mind can't free itself from the worries and anxieties you face during the day, you may find it hard to fall and stay asleep. On top of that, lack of sleep can lead to other problems, including daytime drowsiness, fatigue, and mood swings.

Other health conditions, such as sleep apnea, restless leg syndrome, and insomnia, can also contribute to sleep problems during menopause.

Top Strategies for better sleep

1. Eat well and get plenty of exercise

It's important to eat regular, well-balanced meals that aren't high in fat or sugar and exercise daily to help prevent hot flashes.

The timing of these activities also matters. Eating or exercising too close to bedtime for some people can interrupt the body's natural clock and may inhibit their sleep. Some people find they can sleep better if they exercise in the evening. Experiment and see what works best for you.

2. Wear loose-fitting clothing to bed

Sleep in clothes made from natural fibres, such as cotton. This allows your skin to "breathe" more easily. The fabric helps wick moisture away from your skin.

3. Use cotton sheets

Compared to some other fabrics, cotton stays cooler against your skin. It helps keep heat from building up around you. This can help prevent sweating.

4. Keep your bedroom cool

A cool room is more conducive to sleep than a warm one. Consider lowering the temperature in your home at night. Ceiling fans or standing fans also help circulate air and keep your bedroom cool.

5. Avoid spicy foods

Foods that cause you to sweat may lead to sleep disturbances if you eat them too soon before bedtime. Spicy foods are a common culprit.

6. Avoid nicotine, caffeine, and alcohol

If you drink soda or coffee or smoke too close to bedtime, your body may struggle to counteract the natural boost of energy that caffeine and nicotine give it. A glass of wine before bed may help you fall asleep, but it can interfere with your natural sleep cycle. In other words, you may fall asleep more easily after drinking it, but you're more likely to wake up earlier and feel less rested.

7. Manage your stress

Emotional stress can heighten your sensitivity to temperature changes. This may bring on hot flashes and sweating. Try relaxation techniques such as yoga, exercise, and massage to help manage stress or anxiety that you're facing.

If you feel chronically stressed, anxious, or depressed, speak with your doctor. They may be able to recommend strategies to manage your stress and improve your mood. In some cases, they may prescribe lifestyle changes, medications, or therapy.

8. Take medications as prescribed

If lifestyle treatments aren't effective, your doctor may suggest HRT to help manage your menopause symptoms. Estrogen replacement therapy is most commonly administered through a pill, patch, or vaginal cream. In some cases, estrogen is combined with progesterone.

HRT was once routinely prescribed for hot flashes and other menopause symptoms. However, research now suggests that HRT can raise your risk of certain health conditions, such as:

- blood clots
- stroke
- heart disease
- breast cancer

Ask your doctor about the potential benefits and risks of HRT and other options. There are

medications that are not hormones that have been shown to help women with the symptoms of menopause. Your doctor can help you learn which treatment choices may be best for you.
Loss of sleep can leave you feeling tired, confused, and irritable during the day. It can also raise your risk of accidental injuries and certain health conditions. If hot flashes or other menopause-related symptoms are keeping you awake, speak with your doctor.

Your doctor will probably recommend lifestyle changes to help improve the quality of your sleep. For example, they may encourage you to exercise regularly, adjust your diet, or avoid stimulants before bed. They may also recommend changes to your bedroom environment or sleep routine. In some cases, they may recommend medications, including hormone replacement therapy.

Someone to listen to is an amazing man called Tom Coleman. Tom is a sleep expert based in Ireland and is a fountain of knowledge when it comes to sleep, check out @tomcoleman.ie for his amazing information.

HRT

Hormone replacement therapy (HRT) is a treatment to relieve symptoms of the menopause. It replaces hormones that are at a lower level as you approach the menopause.

The number of American women who take

medication to manage menopause plunged after 2002. That's when news came out that hormone replacement therapy (HRT) could increase the risk of breast cancer, heart disease, stroke, and blood clots.

Yet major medical organizations like the Endocrine Society, North American Menopause Society (NAMS), and the American College of Obstetricians and Gynaecologists (ACOG) say that HRT offers more benefits than risks for many women.

The best approach is to ask your gynaecologist to evaluate the risks and benefits and ask the questions that you want as every woman is different.

Beyond hot flashes, a dry vagina after menopause can make sex painful or cause urination problems. Estrogen applied directly to the vagina, which doesn't pose any risks, helps.

Benefits of HRT:

The main benefit of HRT is that it can help relieve most of the menopausal symptoms, such as:
- hot flushes
- night sweats
- mood swings
- vaginal dryness
- reduced sex drive

Many of these symptoms pass after a few years, but they can be unpleasant and taking HRT can offer relief for many women.

It can also help prevent weakening of the bones (osteoporosis), which is more common after menopause.

Like anything though there can be risks for HRT.

Risks of HRT

The benefits of HRT usually outweigh the risks for most women.

The risks are usually very small, and depend on the type of HRT you take, how long you take it and your own health risks.

Speak to a GP if you're thinking about starting HRT or you're already taking it, and you're worried about any risks.

Breast cancer

There is little or no change in the risk of breast cancer if you take estrogen-only HRT.
Combined HRT can be associated with a small increase in the risk of breast cancer.
The increased risk is related to how long you take HRT, and it falls after you stop taking it.

Because of the risk of breast cancer, it's especially important to attend all your breast cancer screening appointments if you're taking HRT.

Blood clots

The evidence shows that:

- there's no increased risk of blood clots from HRT patches or gels
- taking HRT tablets can increase your risk of blood clots - but this risk is still small

Heart disease and strokes

HRT does not significantly increase the risk of cardiovascular disease (including heart disease and strokes) when started before 60 years of age, and may reduce your risk.

Taking HRT tablets is associated with a small increase in the risk of stroke, but the risk of stroke for women under age 60 is generally very low, so the overall risk is still small.

How to get started on HRT

Speak to a GP if you're interested in starting HRT.

You can usually begin HRT as soon as you start experiencing menopausal symptoms and will not usually need to have any tests first.

A GP can explain the different types of HRT available and help you choose one that's suitable for you.

You'll usually start with a low dose, which may be increased at a later stage. It may take a few weeks to feel the effects of treatment and there may be some side effects at first.

A GP will usually recommend trying treatment for 3 months to see if it helps. If it does not, they may suggest changing your dose, or changing the type of HRT you're taking.

Who can take HRT?

Most women can have HRT if they're having symptoms associated with the menopause.

But HRT may not be suitable if you:

- have a history of breast cancer, ovarian cancer or womb cancer
- have a history of blood clots
- have untreated high blood pressure – your blood pressure will need to be controlled before you can start HRT
- have liver disease
- are pregnant – it's still possible to get pregnant while taking HRT, so you should use contraception until 2 years after your last period if you're under 50, or for 1 year after the age of 50

In these circumstances, alternatives to HRT may be recommended instead.

What hormones are in HRT?

HRT replaces the hormones that a woman's body

no longer produces because of the menopause.

The 2 main hormones used in HRT are:

- *Estrogen* – types used include estradiol, estrone and estriol
- *Progestin* – either a synthetic version of the hormone progesterone (such as dydrogesterone, medroxyprogesterone, norethisterone and levonorgestrel), or a version called micronised progesterone (sometimes called body identical, or natural) that is chemically identical to the human hormone

HRT involves either taking both of these hormones (combined HRT) or just taking estrogen (estrogen-only HRT).

Estrogen-only HRT is usually only recommended if you have had your womb removed during a hysterectomy.

Ways of taking HRT

HRT comes in several different forms. Talk to a GP about the pros and cons of each option.

Tablets

Tablets are 1 of the most common forms of HRT. They are usually taken once a day.

Both estrogen-only and combined HRT are available

as tablets. For some women this may be the simplest way of having treatment.

However, it's important to be aware that some of the risks of HRT, such as blood clots, are higher with tablets than with other forms of HRT (although the overall risk is still small).

Skin patches

Skin patches are also a common way of taking HRT. You stick them to your skin and replace them every few days.

Estrogen-only and combined HRT patches are available.

Skin patches may be a better option than tablets if you find it inconvenient to take a tablet every day.

Using patches can also help avoid some side effects of HRT, such as indigestion, and unlike tablets, they do not increase your risk of blood clots.

Estrogen gel

Estrogen gel is an increasingly popular form of HRT. It's rubbed onto your skin once a day.

Like skin patches, gel can be a convenient way of taking HRT and does not increase your risk of blood clots.

But if you still have your womb, you'll need to take some form of progestogen separately too, to reduce your risk of womb cancer.

Implants

HRT also comes as small pellet-like implants that are inserted under your skin (usually in the tummy area) after your skin has been numbed with local anaesthetic.

The implant releases estrogen gradually and lasts for several months before needing to be replaced.

This may be a convenient option if you do not want to worry about taking your treatment every day or every few days. But if you still have your womb, you'll need to take progestogen separately too.

If you're taking a different form of estrogen and need to take progestogen alongside it, another implant option is the intrauterine system (IUS). An IUS releases a progestogen hormone into the womb. It can stay in place for 3 to 5 years and also acts as a contraceptive.
Implants of HRT are not widely available and are not used very often.

Vaginal estrogen

Estrogen is also available as a cream, pessary or ring that is placed inside your vagina.
This can help relieve vaginal dryness, but will not help with other symptoms such as hot flushes.

It does not carry the usual risks of HRT and does not increase your risk of breast cancer, so you can use it without taking progestogen, even if you still have a womb.

Testosterone

Testosterone is available as a gel that you rub onto your skin. It is not currently licensed for use in women, but it can be prescribed after the menopause by a specialist doctor if they think it might help restore your sex drive.

Testosterone is usually only recommended for women whose low sex drive (libido) does not improve after using HRT. It is used alongside another type of HRT.

Possible side effects of using testosterone include acne and unwanted hair growth.

Ask a GP for more information on testosterone products.

HRT treatment routines

Your treatment routine for HRT depends on whether you're in the early stages of the menopause or have had menopausal symptoms for some time.

The 2 types of routines are cyclical (or sequential) HRT and continuous combined HRT.

Cyclical HRT

Cyclical HRT, also known as sequential HRT, is often recommended for women taking combined HRT who have menopausal symptoms but still have their periods.

There are 2 types of cyclical HRT:

- *monthly HRT* – you take estrogen every day, and take progestogen alongside it for the last 14 days of your menstrual cycle
- *3-monthly HRT* – you take estrogen every day, and take progestogen alongside it for around 14 days every 3 months

Monthly HRT is usually recommended for women having regular periods.

3-monthly HRT is usually recommended for women having irregular periods. You should have a period every 3 months.

It's useful to maintain regular periods so you know when your periods naturally stop and when you're likely to progress to the last stage of the menopause.

Continuous combined HRT

Continuous combined HRT is usually recommended for women who are postmenopausal. A woman is usually said to be postmenopausal if she has not had a period for 1 year.

Continuous combined HRT involves taking oestrogen and progestogen every day without a break.

Estrogen-only HRT is also usually taken every day without a break.

When to stop taking HRT?

There's no limit on how long you can take HRT, but talk to a GP about how long they recommend you take the treatment.

Most women stop taking it once their menopausal symptoms pass, which is usually after a few years.

Women who take HRT for more than 1 year have a higher risk of breast cancer than women who never use HRT. The risk is linked to all types of HRT except vaginal estrogen.

The increased risk of breast cancer falls after you stop taking HRT, but some increased risk remains for more than 10 years compared to women who have never used HRT.

When you decide to stop, you can choose to do so suddenly or gradually.

Gradually decreasing your HRT dose is usually recommended because it's less likely to cause your symptoms to come back in the short term.

Contact a GP if you have symptoms that persist for several months after you stop HRT, or if you have particularly severe symptoms. You may need to start HRT again.

Side effects of HRT

As with any medicine, HRT can cause side effects. But these will usually pass within 3 months of starting treatment.

Common side effects include:

- breast tenderness
- headaches
- feeling sick
- indigestion
- abdominal (tummy) pain
- vaginal bleeding

Alternatives to HRT

If you're unable to take HRT or decide not to, you may want to consider alternative ways of controlling your menopausal symptoms.

What about the risk of Cancer?

Does HRT increase the risk of breast cancer?

Most types of HRT increase the risk of breast cancer. But the risk is higher for those using combined HRT, which uses both estrogen and progestogen.

Vaginal estrogens are not linked to an increased risk of breast cancer, whereas tibolone is.

Taking HRT for 1 year or less only slightly increases breast cancer risk. However, the longer you take HRT the greater the risks are, and the longer they last.

The risk of breast cancer due to HRT can also vary from person to person. Things such as what age you are when you first start taking HRT, other medicines you may be taking, and your general health can impact the risk. If you have a family history of breast cancer or cancer in general you will need to declare this to your doctor as this may put you at further risk.

People who begin HRT before or soon after the menopause may have a bigger risk than those who start HRT later.

Does HRT increase the risk of ovarian cancer?

Yes, both estrogen-only and combined HRT slightly increase the risk of ovarian cancer. But when HRT is stopped, the risk starts to go back to what it would have been if HRT wasn't taken.

It's not yet clear if there's any link between ovarian cancer and tibolone.

Does HRT increase the risk of womb (endometrial) cancer?

The risk of womb cancer depends on the type of HRT.

Estrogen-only HRT increases the risk of womb cancer. The longer this type of HRT is used, the bigger the risk. That's why estrogen-only HRT is usually only offered to those who have had their womb removed (a hysterectomy) as they have no risk of womb cancer to begin with.

Combined HRT can reduce womb cancer risk. But combined treatment causes the biggest increase in breast cancer risk. So, it's important to talk to your doctor about the balance of possible benefits and risks for you.

Similar to estrogen-only HRT, tibolone also increases the risk of womb cancer.

Going on HRT is a personal choice and no one can make you go on it. Like everything else there are pros and cons to taking it. It is important that you know all of your options so please discuss these with your doctor. If you have any underlying health issues or cancer is in the family, please discuss your options further.

Managing the Mind during Menopause

Many women have additional symptoms during both perimenopause and menopause and one of those is the impact it can play on mood. This time in a woman's life is a period of change and this can have an impact on overall mental health.

Perimenopause is the period before menopause when all the symptoms occur. As your reproductive hormone levels change, your body may react with hot flashes, sleep interruptions, and changes in mood that can be unpredictable. Sometimes these mood changes take the form of extreme and sudden feelings of panic, anxiety, or anger.

Feeling anger can be a result of factors connected to menopause. The realities of getting older and moving into a different phase of life — in addition to the stress that lost sleep and hot flashes sometimes cause — can contribute to moods that are unstable. Remember that your body is changing, but you aren't to blame for these emotions. A very real chemical reaction is at play.
Menopause affects all women differently, so it's hard to say how rare or common menopause anger is. Hormone changes can have a significant effect on your mood, but that doesn't mean that you've permanently lost control over the way you feel.

The impact of Estrogen, serotonin, and mood

Estrogen is the hormone that manages most of a woman's reproductive functions. As you approach menopause, your ovaries slow their production of estrogen.

Estrogen also controls how much serotonin is being produced in your brain. Serotonin is a chemical that helps regulate your moods. If you're producing less estrogen, you're also producing less serotonin. This can have a direct impact on how stable and optimistic you feel.

Balancing your hormones is the key to regaining mood control. There are several activities and lifestyle change you can try that might work to balance your hormones naturally.

1. Eat a balanced diet

Your diet has a significant impact on your hormone levels. Adding foods that are rich in vitamin D, calcium, and iron will not only help you feel better, but also keep your bones strong as your estrogen production slows down.

Menopause can be linked to weight gain, which can in turn affect your self-image and your moods. Stick to a high-fiber diet to protect your colon health and keep your digestion regular. Be active. Take the responsibility of caring for your body. Celebrate being able to move your body.

Ongoing research also suggests that plant estrogens found in soy may help reduce menopause symptoms, so consider making edamame, tofu, and soy milk into pantry staples. Women with a medical history of cancer should talk to their doctors before increasing soy in their diet.

Caffeine has been linked to aggravating hot flashes and night sweats, so cutting back here may also be helpful. My advice is no caffeine after 2pm. Drink cool fluids. Sleep with a fan at night.

2. Exercise regularly

Exercise can stimulate endorphin hormones, which boost your mood. Post menopause, you are at an elevated risk for heart disease, so getting some cardio in now is as important as ever for your long-term health.

Low-impact cardiovascular exercise — such as Pilates, elliptical machines, and jogging — can get your blood pumping and improve the way you feel about your body.

The Centres for Disease Control and Prevention (CDC) recommends 150 minutes of moderate cardiovascular exercise per week for older adults, including women in menopause.

3. Channel that anger into creative activity

According to researchers in one clinical trial, perceived control over your symptoms may be an indicator of symptom severity. That could be why some women find it helpful to channel their strong emotions into a productive outlet.

Activities like painting, writing, gardening, and even home decorating can give you the space to process your emotions in a positive way. Support groups or even chats with friends can also be really helpful as sharing your story can help you realise that you are not alone.

When you're able to accept that you're moving into a new phase of life and decide to embrace that change as a positive one, you may see a decrease in your strong mood swings.

4. Practice mindfulness, meditation, and stress management

Mindfulness and meditation can help you regain a positive awareness and feeling of control over your symptoms. Be in the moment. Focus on what your senses are telling you right now. What do you see, smell, feel, hear, taste?

Studies are emerging to probe the effect of mindfulness on depression and anxiety, but we already know that these practices give us a sense of self-compassion and empathy.

By using a mindfulness app, doing deep breathing techniques, or simply starting your day with 10 minutes of free time to think, you're already on your way to a mindfulness practice. One tool that works amazingly with clients is trying to get daily light exposure first thing in the morning. This can help to improve mood, even if it is for as little as 10 minutes.

Use this ability to empty your mind of negative thoughts when your anger flares up. Connect to your feelings deeply during heated moments or uncomfortable hot flashes. The more you practice this habit, the more automatic it will become.

Try journaling —that is, writing out your frustrations. Reflect back on your own behaviour and think of things that were triggers.

Next time an outburst might be prevented by recognizing you're on the path to one. Stop, breathe five deep breaths. Remove yourself from the situation.

When to see your doctor

If you become concerned about the way your mood is affecting your life, make an appointment with your general practitioner or OB-GYN.

You may benefit from targeted treatment if you:

- feel like your behaviour is erratic
- are experiencing panic attacks or insomnia
- have relationships that are suffering as a result of your moods

You should also see your doctor if you're experiencing symptoms of depression. This includes:

- exhaustion
- apathy
- Helplessness

Don't hesitate to involve your doctor. They can help you feel like your usual self again by developing a treatment plan suited to your individual needs.

Treatment options

Your doctor might recommend prescription drugs to help you stabilize your moods.

For example, hormone therapy with low-dose synthetic estrogen is a good choice for some women to help provide symptom relief. Low-dose antidepressants (SSRIs) can help decrease hot flashes and mood swings.

Your doctor might also recommend that you see a psychologist or licensed counsellor to make a mental health plan that addresses your long-term needs. CBT could also be a great option.

If your doctor has suggested going on medication you need to be open and honest about how you feel about this. Some may not feel comfortable about going on medication and no one can make you. Please try to communicate any concerns that you may have and discuss through all your options.

The Menopause Brain Fog

Many women also report feeling forgetful or having a general "brain fog" that makes it hard to concentrate.

Are memory issues part of menopause? Yes. And this "brain fog" is more common than you might think.

What does the research say?

In one study, researchers share that some 60 percent of middle-aged women report difficulty concentrating and other issues with cognition. These issues spike in women going through perimenopause.

The women in the study noticed subtle changes in memory, but the researchers also believe that a "negative effect" may have made these feelings more pronounced.

The researchers explain that women going through menopause may generally feel a more negative mood, and that mood may be related to memory issues. Not only that, but "brain fog" may also be connected with sleep issues and vascular symptoms associated with menopause, like hot flashes.

Another study also focuses on the idea that women in early stages of menopause may experience more noticeable issues with cognition. Specifically, women in the first year of their last menstrual period scored the lowest on tests evaluating:

- verbal learning
- memory
- motor function
- attention
- working memory tasks

Memory for the women improved over time, which is the opposite of what the researchers had initially hypothesized.
What's causing this foggy thinking?

Scientists believe it has something to do with hormone changes. Estrogen, progesterone, follicle stimulating hormone, and luteinizing hormone are all responsible for different processes in the body, including cognition. Perimenopause lasts an average of 4 years, during which time your hormone levels may fluctuate wildly and cause a range of symptoms as the body and mind adjust.

Seeking help

Memory issues during menopause can be completely normal. You may forget where you placed your phone or have trouble remembering an acquaintance's name. If your cognitive issues are starting to negatively impact your daily life, however, it may be time to see your doctor just to make sure it is not dementia or Alzheimer's.

Treatment

Once your doctor has ruled out other issues, like dementia, you may explore menopausal hormone therapy (MHT). This treatment involves taking either low-dose estrogen or a combination of estrogen and progestin. These hormones may help with the many symptoms you experience during menopause, not just memory loss.

Long-term use of estrogen may increase your risk of breast cancer, cardiovascular disease, and other health issues. Speak with your doctor about the benefits versus the risks of this type of treatment.

Prevention

You may not be able to prevent the "brain fog" associated with menopause. Still, there are some lifestyle changes you can make that may ease your symptoms and improve your memory overall.

<u>Eat a well-balanced diet</u>

A diet that's high in low-density lipoprotein (LDL) cholesterol and fat may not be ideal for both your heart and your brain. Instead, try filling up on whole foods and healthy fats.

The Mediterranean diet, for example, may help with brain health because it's rich in omega-3 fatty acids and other unsaturated fats.

A diet that includes some of these foods could be very beneficial:

- fresh fruits and vegetables
- whole grains
- fish
- beans and nuts
- olive oil

<u>Get enough rest</u>

Your sleep quality may make your "brain fog" worse. With sleep problems high on the list of symptoms associated with menopause, getting enough rest can be a tall order. In fact, some 61 percent of postmenopausal women report insomnia issues.

What you can do:

- *Avoid eating large meals before bedtime.* And steer clear of spicy or acidic foods. They may cause hot flashes.
- *Skip stimulants like caffeine and nicotine before bed.* Alcohol may also disrupt your sleep.
- *Dress for success.* Don't wear heavy clothing or pile on lots of blankets in bed. Turning down the thermostat or using a fan may help keep you cool.
- *Work on relaxation.* Stress can make snoozing even more difficult. Try deep breathing, yoga, or massage.

Exercise your body

Getting regular physical activity is recommended for all people, including women going through menopause. Researchers believe that exercise may even help with symptoms like memory issues.

What you can do:

- Try getting 30 minutes of cardiovascular exercise at least five days a week for a total of 150 minutes. Activities to try include walking, jogging, cycling or any movement that you enjoy.
- Incorporate strength training into your routine as well. Try lifting free weights or using weight machines at your gym at least twice/three times a week.

Exercise your mind

Your brain needs regular workouts as you age. Try doing crossword puzzles, sudoku or starting a new hobby, like playing the piano. Getting out socially may help as well. Even keeping a list of the things, you need to do in the day may help you organize your mind when you're feeling foggy.

Memory and other cognitive issues associated with menopause may improve with time. Eat well, get good sleep, exercise, and keep your mind active to help with your symptoms in the meantime.

If your "brain fog" gets worse, make an appointment with your doctor to rule out other health issues or to ask about hormone treatments for menopause.

What about headaches/migraines?

Menopause can affect your headaches in several ways. The effects can be different for every woman, so you may not experience the same changes as someone else.

If your headaches are hormonal in nature, you may find relief after menopause. This may mean that you have less headaches or less severe headaches. This is because your hormone levels stay low, with little fluctuation, after your period stops for good.

On the other hand, some women have more frequent or worse headaches during perimenopause. It's even possible for women who have never had problems with hormonal headaches to start having headaches during this time.

Women who experience migraines often report that their headaches are significantly worse during perimenopause.

Migraines are a subtype of headache. They're typically the most debilitating in nature. They're characterized by throbbing pain on one side of the head, as well as sensitivity to light or sound.

Estrogen withdrawal is a common trigger. This is why headaches can be worse around menstruation. The same hormone — or lack thereof — that gives some women relief from migraines after menopause can cause more headaches in the months leading up to it.

That's because hormone levels such as estrogen and progesterone decline during perimenopause. This decline isn't always consistent, so women who experience headaches related to their monthly menstrual cycle may have more headaches during perimenopause. It's also common to experience more severe headaches during this time.

Does this mean hormone therapy can affect your headaches?

Your doctor may prescribe some form of hormone replacement therapy (HRT) to treat hot flashes or other symptoms related to menopause. How this treatment affects your headaches will be unique to you. It could help your migraines, or it could make them worse.

If you've noticed worsening headaches and are on HRT, you should tell your doctor. They may want you to try an estrogen skin patch instead. Estrogen patches may be less likely than other forms of HRT to trigger headaches. Your doctor may also suggest other treatment options.

Looking into taking progesterone-alone could be very beneficial. Progesterone calms the brain and is therefore, one of the best ways to prevent and treat your premenstrual and peri menopausal migraines. Please talk to your doctor to discuss all your options.

How to prevent or alleviate headache pain

A number of medications can help treat or even prevent migraines. Some are available over the counter. Others require a doctor's prescription.

Diet and lifestyle changes can also help to reduce the number of headaches you have or alleviate your symptoms.

Diet changes

What you eat can have a huge impact on your headaches. Keep in mind that what triggers your headaches won't be the same for someone else. Because of this, you may want to keep a food diary to determine what your headache triggers may be.

When you experience a headache, write down what you ate in the hours before. Over time this may help you find dietary patterns. If a pattern emerges, you

should try limiting that item.
From there, you can determine if cutting this out of your diet has an effect on your headaches.

Some of the most common dietary triggers I've seen with clients include:

- alcohol, especially red wine
- aged cheeses, such as Parmesan
- caffeine
- chocolate
- dairy products

Supplementation

Magnesium

According to a 2016 meta-analysis, magnesium is one of the best supplements for migraine prevention. A dose of 100mg -300mg will be the recommendation. Start on a lower dose and increase from there if needed. If you are on any medications please check with your doctor before taking it.

Vitamin b2 (riboflavin)

Vitamin b2 (riboflavin) has been clinically trialled for migraine prevention and found to reduce their frequency and was found to reduce their frequency by 50%. The dosage in the trials was 200mg twice per day.

Vitamin D and Coenzyme Q10 may also be beneficial. Taking ibuprofen short term could help manage the pain too. You should check with your doctor before adding these to your regimen to make sure you're not taking any unnecessary risks.

Exercise

Regular physical activity may also help to prevent headaches. Aim for 30 minutes of exercise three to four times each week. Spinning or swimming classes are two great choices. A nice walk outside is easy and accessible, too.

The fluctuations in strength and energy in your training that you saw when your cycle was regular, may be different on HRT. This will depend on the type of HRT that you are taking. Taking HRT will reduce the hormone fluctuations and therefore increase muscle mass (getting that toned look) and increase strength.

It's important to go slow in your activity goals. Let your body warm up gradually. Jumping into a high-intensity workout right away could actually trigger a headache.

Acupuncture

This is a form of alternative medicine that uses thin needles to stimulate your body's energy pathways. Acupuncture stems from traditional Chinese medicine and is used to treat various types of pain. Views on its effectiveness are mixed, but you may find that it helps you.

CBT

Cognitive behavioural therapy (CBT) is slightly different. CBT teaches you stress relief techniques, as well as how to better deal with stressors or pain. It's often recommended that you pair CBT with biofeedback or relaxation therapy for best results.

Although it's not guaranteed, menopause can bring many women relief from headaches once the hormonal roller coaster has officially stopped. Until then, you should work with your doctor to find the best combination of medications or lifestyle changes for you.

If you notice your headaches are becoming worse or interfering with your quality of life, you should speak with your doctor. They can rule out any other causes and, if necessary, adjust your treatment plan.

What about Bone health?

As women enter menopause, their estrogen and progesterone levels begin to fall. Estrogen acts as a natural protector and defender of bone strength. The lack of estrogen contributes to the development of osteoporosis or osteopenia.

Decreased estrogen levels aren't the only cause for osteoporosis.

Other factors may be responsible for weakened bones. When these factors are combined with decreased estrogen levels during menopause, osteoporosis may begin or develop faster if it's already occurring in your bones.

What is Osteoporosis?

Osteoporosis is a disease that causes bone tissue to thin and become less dense. This produces weakened bones that are more susceptible to fracture.

Osteopenia can be considered the first step toward osteoporosis. Technically, it's just a way of saying that your bone density is lower than normal, but not yet causing real problems.

Osteoporosis shows very few symptoms and can progress to advanced stages without presenting any problems. So, it's often not discovered until your weakened bones fracture or break. Once you have a fracture as a result of osteoporosis, you're more susceptible to another.

These breaks can be debilitating. Most often, your weakened bones aren't discovered until after a catastrophic fall that results in a broken hip or back. These injuries can leave you with limited or no mobility for several weeks or months. Surgery may also be required for treatment.

How does Osteoporosis develop?

The exact cause of Osteoporosis is unknown. However, we do know how the disease develops and what it does to your bones.

Think of your bones as living, growing, and ever-changing entities of your body. Imagine the outer part of your bone as a case. Inside the case is a more delicate bone with little holes in it, similar to a sponge.

If you fall when your bones are in this state, they may not be strong enough to sustain the fall, and they'll fracture. If osteoporosis is severe, fractures can occur even without a fall or other trauma.

The following are additional risk factors for osteoporosis:

- Age
- Smoking
- Body composition
- Existing bone density
- Family history
- Gender
- Race and ethnicity

How to get a diagnosis?

Since osteopenia usually develops without symptoms, you may not know that your bones are becoming weaker until you begin to have serious problems or the condition progresses to osteoporosis.

A primary care physician may screen you for your risk of osteopenia and osteoporosis.

Bone density tests are usually done with dual-energy X-ray absorptiometry (DXA/DEXA) scans of the hip and lower spine.

This testing is also recommended for:

- women over age 65
- women under age 65 who have evidence of lower bone mass
- men over age 70
- men over age 50 with certain risk factors for bone loss

BMD measurements and your FRAX (Fracture Risk Assessment Tool) score are usually used together to get an idea of your overall bone health and guide treatment.

Treatment options

Take calcium and vitamin D supplements

Calcium can help build strong bones and keep them strong as you age. The National Institutes of Health (NIH)Trusted Source recommends that people ages 19 to 50 get 1,000 milligrams (mg) of calcium each day.

Women over 50 and all adults over 70 should get at least 1,200 mg of calcium each day.

If you can't get adequate calcium through food sources like dairy products, kale, and broccoli, talk with your doctor about supplements. Both calcium carbonate and calcium citrate deliver good forms of calcium to your body.

Vitamin D is important for healthy bones, as your body can't properly absorb calcium without it. Fatty fishes like salmon or mackerel are good sources of vitamin D from food, along with foods like milk and cereals in which vitamin D is added.

Sun exposure is the natural way the body makes vitamin D. But the time it takes in the sun to produce vitamin D varies depending on time of day, the environment, where you live, and the natural pigment of your skin. If you are living in a climate similar to Ireland and the UK all of us should be supplementing with Vitamin D between the months of October and March.

For people concerned with skin cancer or for those who wish to get their vitamin D in other ways, supplements are available.

According to the NIH, people ages 19 to 70 should get at least 600 international units (IU) of vitamin D every day. People over 70 should increase their daily vitamin D to 800 IU.

Ask your doctor about prescription medications and injectable bone-building agents
A group of drugs called bisphosphonates helps prevent bone loss. Over time, these medicines have been shown to slow bone loss, increase bone density, and reduce the risk of bone fractures.

A 2017 study showed bisphosphonates can reduce the rate of fractures due to osteoporosis up to 60 percent.

Monoclonal antibodies can also be used to help prevent bone loss. These drugs include denosumab and romosozumab (Evenity).

Selective estrogen receptor modulators, or SERMs, are a group of drugs that have estrogen-like properties. They're sometimes used for the prevention and treatment of osteoporosis.

A 2016 study showed that the most benefit in SERMS is often in reducing the risk of fractures in the spine up to 42 percent.

Resistance Training

Exercise often does as much for building and maintaining strong bones as medication does. Unfortunately, there is a common myth that women will get bulky if they lift weights, this is not the case. Women have not got enough testosterone in their bodies for this to occur. If you are looking for that toned (real name gaining muscle) look at lifting weights 2 to 3 times per week.

Talk to your doctor about hormone replacement therapy

Hormone replacement therapy (HRT) can help prevent bone loss caused by the decreased levels of estrogen that occurs during perimenopause and menopause. However, experts currently recommend that HRT be used only after other options for bone health have been considered.

HRT may have a role when treating other symptoms

of menopause, including hot flashes, night sweats, and mood swings. However, this therapy isn't for everyone. It may not be the correct treatment option if you have a personal history of or are at an increased risk for:

Bone loss is a natural part of aging, but there are some things — like gender and diet — that can speed the process along.

If your bone density is lower than normal, you may be diagnosed with osteopenia. While this is not quite osteoporosis, the condition is still serious.

With osteopenia, you have time to make changes that can protect your bone health. If your condition has advanced to osteoporosis, talk to your doctor about what you can do to preserve your bone strength and prevent additional loss

Sex life and menopause

As you go through menopause, you might notice that your libido, or sex drive, is changing. Some women may experience an increase in libido, while others experience a decrease.

Menopause can negatively affect libido in several ways. During menopause, your testosterone and estrogen levels both decrease, which may make it more difficult for you to get aroused.

A decrease in estrogen can also lead to vaginal dryness. Lower levels of estrogen lead to a drop in blood supply in the vagina, which can then negatively affect vaginal lubrication. It can also lead to thinning of the vaginal wall, known as vaginal atrophy. Vaginal dryness and atrophy often lead to discomfort during sex.

Other physical changes during menopause might also affect your libido. For example, many women gain weight during menopause, and discomfort with your new body can decrease your desire for sex. Hot flashes and night sweats are also common symptoms. These symptoms can leave you feeling too tired for sex. Other symptoms include mood symptoms, such as depression and irritability, which can turn you off from sex.

See your doctor if you're going through menopause and noticing changes in your libido, your doctor can help determine the underlying cause of those changes. In preparation for the chat with your doctor I would recommend making notes on any concerns you have, write down any questions that you may have and before the consultation say that you may be nervous.

Some of the things that can help include:

- Lubricant
- Exercise
- Communication with partner
- HRT
- Kegel exercises
- Therapy

Sex life can be a difficult time as you are going through peri menopause and menopause so it's important to know that you are not alone on this. Others have got through this and you will too. Sex doesn't have to be awkward knowing how your body works and making it work for you can be liberating.

Conclusion

Menopause can be challenging, both physically and emotionally.

However, eating a nutritious diet and getting enough exercise, sleep and stress management can help prevent weight gain and reduce disease risk.

Although it may take some time to adjust to the processes taking place in your body, try to do your best to accept these changes that will inevitably happen with age.
Women spend one third of their life after menopause so life really starts after. The journey so far has been to listen and now you can look forward to living a life that you want and start to do things that you may never have thought about doing.

Perimenopause and menopause are both transitional phases in a woman's life that indicate an end to your reproductive years.

There are certainly adjustments to be made, but remember that not all aspects are negative. Remember that you are going to spend over a third of your life after this stage so it really is the start of something rather beautiful rather than something to mourn.

Chapter 9 - Thyroid

What is a thyroid gland?

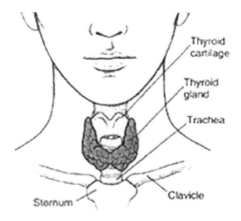

The thyroid gland is an endocrine gland in your neck. The thyroid gland is a small butterfly-shaped gland in the neck, just in front of the windpipe (trachea). It makes two hormones that are secreted into the blood: thyroxine (T4) and triiodothyronine (T3). These hormones are necessary for all the cells in your body to work normally.

Thyroid disorders are very common and tend mainly to occur in women, although anybody - men, teenagers, children, and babies, too - can be affected. About one in 20 people has some kind of thyroid disorder, which may be temporary or permanent.

The thyroid gland lies in the front of your neck in a position just below your Adam's apple. It is made up of two lobes - the right lobe and the left lobe, each about the size of a plum cut in half - and these two lobes are joined by a small bridge of thyroid tissue called the isthmus. The two lobes lie on either side of your windpipe.

What do my thyroid hormones do for you?

The T4, or rather the T3 derived from it, and the T3 regulates the speed with which your body cells work. If too much of the thyroid hormones are secreted, the body cells work faster than normal, and you have hyperthyroidism. If you become hyperthyroid because of too much secretion of the hormones from the thyroid gland, the increased activity of your body cells or body organs may lead, for example, to a quickening of your heart rate or increased activity of your intestine so that you have frequent bowel motions or even diarrhoea.

On the other hand, if too little of the thyroid hormones are produced (known as hypothyroidism), the cells and organs of your body slow down. If you become hypothyroid, your heart rate, for example, may be slower than normal and your intestines work sluggishly, so you become constipated.

<u>Difference between underactive thyroid and overactive thyroid</u>

Hypothyroidism occurs when your body doesn't produce enough thyroid hormones. This is also called underactive thyroid. Hypothyroidism affects women more frequently than men.

If you've recently been diagnosed with

hypothyroidism, it's important to know that treatment is considered simple, safe, and effective and this is what the next few sections are going to go through.

How common is hypothyroidism?

Hypothyroidism is a fairly common condition.

About 4.6 percent of Americans ages 12 years old and up have hypothyroidism. Overall, about 10 million people in the United States live with the condition.

Women are more likely to have an underactive thyroid. In fact, 1 in 8 women will develop hypothyroidism. The disease gets more common with age. People over 60 years old experience it more frequently.

What are the signs and symptoms of hypothyroidism?

The signs and symptoms of hypothyroidism vary from person to person so it is important to keep a log of these so that you can present this to your doctor. This could make diagnosis easier for your GP.

Early symptoms can include weight gain and fatigue. Both become more common as you age, regardless of your thyroid's health. You may not realize that these changes are related to your thyroid until more symptoms appear.

The most common signs and symptoms of

hypothyroidism include:

- fatigue
- weight gain
- puffy, sensitive face
- depression
- constipation
- feeling cold
- decreased sweating
- slowed heart rate
- elevated blood cholesterol
- dry skin
- dry, thinning hair
- impaired memory
- fertility difficulties or menstrual changes
- muscle weakness
- muscle stiffness, aches, and tenderness
- pain and stiffness in your joints
- Hoarseness

For most people, symptoms of the condition progress gradually over many years. As the thyroid slows more and more, the symptoms may become more easily identified. Of course, many of these symptoms also become more common with age in general.

If you suspect your symptoms are the result of a thyroid problem, talk with your doctor. They can order a blood test to determine if you have hypothyroidism.

What causes hypothyroidism?

Hashimoto's thyroiditis

Your immune system is designed to protect your body's cells against invading bacteria and viruses. When unknown bacteria or viruses enter your body, your immune system responds by sending out fighter cells to destroy the foreign cells.

Sometimes, your body confuses normal, healthy cells for invading cells. This is called an autoimmune response. If the autoimmune response isn't regulated or treated, your immune system can attack healthy tissues. This can cause serious medical issues, including conditions such as hypothyroidism.

Hashimoto's thyroiditis is an autoimmune condition and the most common cause of an underactive thyroid in the United States. This disease attacks your thyroid gland and causes chronic thyroid inflammation. The inflammation can reduce thyroid function.

It affects middle-aged women most commonly, but it can occur in men and children. This condition can also have a genetic factor. If a family member has been diagnosed with the disease, then your risk for having it is higher.

Treatment

Treatment for this condition aims to reduce and normalize thyroid hormone production.

Sometimes, treatment can cause the levels of your thyroid hormone to remain low permanently. This often occurs after treatment with radioactive iodine.

Surgical removal of your thyroid
If your entire thyroid gland is removed as a result of thyroid problems, you'll develop hypothyroidism. Using thyroid medication for the rest of your life is the primary treatment.

If only a portion of the gland is removed, your thyroid may still be able to produce enough hormones on its own. Blood tests will help determine how much thyroid medication you'll need.

Radiation therapy

If you've been diagnosed with cancer of the head or neck, lymphoma, or leukaemia, you may have undergone radiation therapy. Radiation used for the treatment of these conditions may slow or halt the production of thyroid hormone. This will almost always lead to hypothyroidism.

Medications

Several medicines may lower thyroid hormone production, leading to hypothyroidism. These include ones used to treat psychological conditions, cancer, or heart disease, such as:

- lithium
- mitotane (Lysodren), an adrenal cancer medication
- interleukin-2 (IL-2)

- amiodarone (Pacerone), an antiarrhythmic drug

What are the risk factors for hypothyroidism?

Factors that can increase your risk of developing hypothyroidism include:

- being female
- being at least 60 years old
- having a family history of hypothyroidism
- having certain autoimmune conditions, such as Sjögren syndrome and type 1 diabetes

How is hypothyroidism diagnosed?

Two primary tools are used to determine if you have hypothyroidism, a medical evaluation and blood tests.

<u>Medical evaluation</u>

Your doctor will complete a thorough physical exam and medical history. They'll check for physical signs of hypothyroidism, including:

- dry skin
- slowed reflexes
- swelling in the neck
- a slower heart rate

In addition, your doctor will ask you to report any symptoms you've been experiencing, such as fatigue, depression, constipation, or constantly feeling cold.

If you have a known family history of thyroid conditions, tell your doctor during this conversation.

Blood tests

Blood tests are the only way to reliably confirm a diagnosis of hypothyroidism.

A thyroid-stimulating hormone (TSH) test measures how much TSH your pituitary gland is creating:

- If your thyroid isn't producing enough hormones, the pituitary gland will boost TSH to increase thyroid hormone production.
- If you have hypothyroidism, your TSH levels will be high, as your body is trying to stimulate more thyroid hormone activity.
- If you have hyperthyroidism, your TSH levels will be low, as your body is trying to stop excessive thyroid hormone production.

A thyroxine (T4) level test is also useful in diagnosing hypothyroidism. T4 is one of the hormones directly produced by your thyroid. Used together, T4 and TSH tests help evaluate thyroid function.

Typically, if you have a low level of T4 along with a high level of TSH, you have hypothyroidism. However, there's a spectrum of thyroid disease. Other thyroid function tests may be necessary to properly diagnose your condition.

Which medications are available to treat hypothyroidism?

Hypothyroidism is a lifelong condition. For many people, medication reduces or alleviates symptoms.

Hypothyroidism is best treated by using levothyroxine (Levoxyl, Synthroid). This synthetic version of the T4 hormone copies the action of the thyroid hormone your body would normally produce.

The medication is designed to return adequate levels of thyroid hormone to your blood. Once hormone levels are restored, symptoms of the condition are likely to disappear or at least become much more manageable.

Once you start treatment, it takes several weeks before you begin feeling relief. You'll require follow-up blood tests to monitor your progress. You and your doctor will work together to find a dose and a treatment plan that best addresses your symptoms. This can take some time.

In most cases, people with hypothyroidism must remain on this medication their entire lives. However, it's unlikely you'll continue to take the same dose, especially if you have Hashimoto's thyroiditis. To make sure your medication is still working properly, your doctor should test your TSH levels regularly.

What about alternative treatments?

Animal extracts that contain thyroid hormone are available. These extracts come from the thyroid glands of pigs. They contain both T4 and triiodothyronine (T3).

If you take levothyroxine, you're only receiving T4. However, that's all you need because your body is capable of producing T3 from the synthetic T4.

These alternative animal extracts often contain inconsistent amounts of each hormone, and studies haven't shown them to be better than levothyroxine. For these reasons, they aren't routinely recommended.

Do tell your doctor if you decide to try to use other products so they can adjust your treatment accordingly.

Other treatments include the likes of Selenium, Vitamin B, or Ashwagandha.

<u>Selenium</u>

According to the National Institutes of Health (NIH), selenium is a trace element that plays a part in thyroid hormone metabolism.

Many foods contain selenium, including:

- tuna
- turkey
- Brazil nuts

- grass-fed beef

Hashimoto's thyroiditis often reduces the body's selenium supply. Supplementing this trace element has shown to help balance thyroxine, or T4, levels in some people.

It's important to talk with your doctor about how much selenium may be right for you since every person is different. Please don't take more than 200 micrograms per day.

Vitamin B

Taking certain vitamin supplements can have an effect on your thyroid health.

Low thyroid hormones can affect your body's vitamin B-12 levels. Taking a vitamin B-12 supplement may help you repair some of the damage hypothyroidism caused.

Vitamin B-12 can help with the tiredness thyroid disease can cause. The disease also affects your vitamin B-1 levels. You can add more B vitamins to your diet with the following foods:

- peas and beans
- asparagus
- sesame seeds
- tuna
- cheese
- milk
- Eggs

Vitamin B-12 is generally safe for most healthy

individuals at recommended levels. Talk with your doctor about how much vitamin B-12 may be right for you.

Ashwagandha

No human studies have examined ashwagandha supplements and hyperthyroidism.

Preliminary research shows that ashwagandha may improve thyroid levels in those with hypothyroidism. However, it may worsen the symptoms of hyperthyroidism. The dosage for this supplement is advised at 300-mg tablets ingested twice per day after eating.

It is important to speak with your healthcare practitioner before taking ashwagandha, especially if you have hyperthyroidism (underactive thyroid).

What about Iodine?

Avoid it as a supplement whether you have hyperthyroidism or hypothyroidism. The effect of iodine supplements can vary by person, causing the thyroid to produce either too much or too little hormone.

You usually don't need iodine supplements if you live in most developed countries. Some alternative medicine specialists suggest iodine tablets or kelp supplements — which are high in iodine — for hypothyroidism. An underactive thyroid (hypothyroidism) occurs when your body doesn't make enough thyroid hormones for your body's needs.

It's true that not having enough iodine (iodine deficiency) can cause hypothyroidism. But iodine deficiency has been rare in the United States and other developed countries since iodine has been added to salt (iodized salt) and other foods.

If the underactive thyroid isn't caused by iodine deficiency, then iodine supplements give no benefit and shouldn't be taken.

In fact, for some people with an underactive thyroid, too much iodine can cause or worsen their condition. Your doctor will be able to guide you on this so please reach out to them for more information.

Hypothyroidism can be safely and effectively treated with a drug — the synthetic thyroid hormone levothyroxine (Synthroid, Levoxyl, others).

What are the complications of hypothyroidism?

Complications of hypothyroidism include:

- goiter (swelling of the thyroid gland that causes a lump in the front of the neck)
- nerve injury
- peripheral neuropathy
- carpal tunnel syndrome
- reduced kidney function, in cases of severe disease
- myxedema coma, in cases of severe disease
- obstructive sleep apnea

Hypothyroidism can also result in infertility or pregnancy-related complications such as preeclampsia.

Nutrition for hypothyroidism

As a general rule, people with hypothyroidism don't have a specific diet they should follow. However, here are some recommendations to keep in mind.

Eat a balanced diet

Your thyroid needs adequate amounts of iodine in order to fully function, but you don't need to take an iodine supplement for that to happen.

A balanced diet of whole grains, beans, lean proteins, and colourful fruits and vegetables should provide enough iodine. Discover other iodine-rich foods.

Monitor your soy intake

Soy may hinder the absorption of thyroid hormones. If you drink or eat too many soy products, you may not be able to properly absorb your medication.

It's especially important that caregivers monitor the soy intake of infants who need hypothyroidism treatment and also drink soy formula.

Soy is found in:

- tofu
- vegan cheese and meat products
- soy milk
- soybeans
- soy sauce

You need steady doses of the medication to achieve even levels of thyroid hormone in your blood. Avoid eating or drinking soy-based foods for at least 4 hours before and after you take your medication.

Be smart with fibre

Like soy, fibre may interfere with hormone absorption. Too much dietary fibre may prevent your body from getting the hormones it needs.

Fibre is vital, so don't avoid it entirely. Instead, avoid taking your medicine within several hours of eating high fibre foods.

Don't take thyroid medication with other supplements

If you take supplements or medications in addition to thyroid medications, try to take them at different times. Other medications can interfere with absorption, so it's best to take your thyroid medication on an empty stomach and without other medications or foods.

Being diagnosed with hypothyroidism doesn't mean you'll have to follow a strict diet, although a few adjustments may be necessary. Create a hypothyroidism diet plan with these tips.

Is there a connection between hypothyroidism and depression?

When levels of thyroid hormones are low, your body's natural functions slow down and lag. This causes a variety of symptoms, including fatigue, weight gain, and even depression. A 2016 study found that 60 percent of people with hypothyroidism exhibited some symptoms of depression.

Some people with hypothyroidism may only experience mood difficulties. This can make diagnosing hypothyroidism difficult. Instead of only treating the brain, doctors should also consider testing for and treating an underactive thyroid.

Depression and hypothyroidism share several symptoms. These include:

- fatigue
- weight gain
- depressed mood
- reduced desire and satisfaction
- difficulty concentrating
- sleep difficulties

The two conditions also have symptoms that may distinguish them from one another. For hypothyroidism, problems such as dry skin, constipation, high cholesterol, and hair loss are common. For depression alone, these conditions wouldn't be expected.

Depression is often a diagnosis made based on

symptoms and medical history. Low thyroid function is diagnosed with a physical exam and blood tests (see the section earlier in the chapter). To see if there's a link between your depression and your thyroid function, your doctor can order these tests for a definitive diagnosis.

If your depression is caused only by hypothyroidism, correcting the hypothyroidism should treat the depression. If it doesn't, your doctor may prescribe medications for both conditions.
They'll slowly adjust your doses until your depression and hypothyroidism come under control.

What's about the connection between hypothyroidism and anxiety?

While hypothyroidism has long been associated with depression, a 2016 study indicates it may be associated with anxiety too.

Researchers evaluated 100 people between the ages of 18 and 45 years old who have a known history of hypothyroidism. Using an anxiety questionnaire, they found that around 63 percent of them met the criteria for some form of anxiety.

Research to date has consisted of small studies. Larger and more focused studies on anxiety may help determine if a true connection exists between hypothyroidism and anxiety.

It's important for you and your doctor to discuss all your symptoms when being evaluated for thyroid conditions.

What's the effect of hypothyroidism on pregnancy?

Women who have hypothyroidism and wish to become pregnant face a particular set of challenges. Low thyroid function or uncontrolled hypothyroidism during pregnancy can cause:

- anaemia
- miscarriage
- preeclampsia
- stillbirth
- low birth weight
- brain development problems
- birth defects

If you have hypothyroidism and are pregnant, it's important to take the following steps during the time you're expecting:

<u>Talk to your doctor about testing</u>

Women can develop hypothyroidism while they're pregnant. Some doctors routinely check thyroid levels during pregnancy to monitor for low thyroid hormone levels. If your levels are lower than they should be, your doctor may suggest treatment.

Some women who never had thyroid problems before they were pregnant may develop them after having a baby. This is called postpartum thyroiditis. For many women, the condition resolves within 12 to 18 months, and medication is no longer required.

Approximately 20 percent of women with postpartum thyroiditis will go on to require long-term therapy.

Stay up to date with your medication

Continue to take your medication as prescribed. It's common to have frequent testing so your doctor can make any necessary adjustments to your thyroid medication as your pregnancy progresses. This ensures that the baby is getting enough thyroid hormone for organ development.

Eat well

Your body needs more nutrients, vitamins, and minerals while you're pregnant. Eating a well-balanced diet and taking multivitamins while pregnant can help you maintain a healthy pregnancy.

Women with thyroid problems can and very often do have healthy pregnancies.

You should talk to your doctor if you're trying to get pregnant and have underlying thyroid (both underactive and overactive) or autoimmune disease or prior pregnancy complications. Your doctor can order the appropriate tests and develop a healthy pregnancy plan. The earlier you can prepare, the better your chances are for a successful outcome. And don't underestimate the importance of exercising regularly, eating healthily, and reducing your stress levels.

What about perimenopause and menopause and

thyroid issues?

Hypothyroidism and menopause share some symptoms. Hypothyroidism is also most common in middle-aged women. It's at this time that women are going through menopause. Please check out the chapter on perimenopause and menopause for more information.

Estrogen levels significantly decrease during menopause. This causes many of the symptoms associated with menopause. Estrogen levels may also affect thyroid function.

Hypothyroidism can increase or worsen symptoms of menopause. A research study from 2007 showed that women with a thyroid disorder and severe menopause experienced improved symptoms after getting treated for the thyroid disorder. This suggests that treating thyroid disorders can help manage menopause symptoms.

Thyroid disorders may also increase your risk for long-term complications of menopause. One of the most common complications of menopause is osteoporosis, or loss of bone density.

Another common complication of menopause is increased risk of cardiovascular diseases. Low levels of thyroid hormones also increase risk of heart disorders.

Talk to your doctor if you suspect thyroid issues or if you're experiencing menopause symptoms. Your primary care doctor may refer you to an endocrinologist. The same tests as mentioned above will be run and these include a TSH test, T4 test, T3 Test, TSI test.

Hypothyroidism and menopause share some symptoms. Research also indicates levels of estrogen may impact levels of thyroid hormones. Other research suggests that hypothyroidism can increase symptoms and complications of menopause. You may experience symptoms such as fatigue and weight changes. If these symptoms are persistent, talk to your doctor and provide them with detailed information about your symptoms and menstrual cycle.

What's the connection between hypothyroidism and weight gain?

Your thyroid is responsible for many of your body's daily functions, including metabolism, organ function, and temperature control. When your body doesn't produce enough thyroid hormone, all of these functions can slow down.

If your thyroid gland doesn't function properly, your basal metabolic rate may be low. For that reason, an underactive thyroid is commonly associated with weight gain. The more severe the condition is, the greater your weight gain is likely to be.

The typical amount of weight gain isn't very high, though. Most people will gain somewhere between 5 and 10 pounds.

Properly treating the condition can help you lose any

weight you gained while your thyroid levels were uncontrolled. So once your medication is at the correct dose it is still possible to lose weight. That is why it is essential you attend your check-ups with your doctor.
However, keep in mind that that's not always the case.

It's not uncommon for people with low thyroid hormone levels to lose no weight after they're treated for the condition. That doesn't mean the condition isn't being properly treated. Instead, it may indicate that your weight gain was the result of lifestyle choices rather than low hormone levels.

I have seen many clients with thyroid concerns see amazing rules and live an amazing life once the correct medication and treatment has been provided by your doctor.

What's the connection between hypothyroidism and weight loss?

Once you're treated for this condition, you may lose any weight that you've gained. That's because once your thyroid levels are restored, your ability to manage your weight returns to normal.

If you're treating hypothyroidism but don't see a change in your weight, that doesn't mean weight loss is impossible. Work with a doctor, registered dietitian, or nutritionist to create a routine that will work for.

Exercise and Hypothyroidism

Hypothyroidism, or having an underactive thyroid, can cause many symptoms like fatigue, joint pain, heart palpitations, and depression. The condition also reduces overall metabolism, making those with hypothyroidism more prone to weight gain, if medication is not dosed correctly.

Having low levels of thyroid hormones can reduce cardiac fitness. Regularly participating in activities like running, walking at a brisk pace, or playing a sport can improve cardiac health. The related mood-boosting benefits can also relieve other hypothyroidism symptoms including depression and fatigue.

Building muscle (or getting toned) can also help. Because hypothyroidism lowers your body's resting metabolic rate, people with this condition are more liable to gain weight and suffer secondary problems caused by obesity. Building muscle through strength training can counteract these effects.

If you are someone who suffers with joint pain, light walking, yoga or cycling may help. Always seek guidance if you are going under a new exercise program.

So, we have looked into an underactive thyroid (hypothyroidism). Now it's important to look into an overactive thyroid (hyperthyroidism) and understand what the difference is, the symptoms, diagnosis, and how to manage it through diet and lifestyle.

What is hyperthyroidism (over active thyroid)?

As mentioned before your thyroid gland regulates your metabolism through the release of these hormones. An overactive thyroid, also known as hyperthyroidism or thyrotoxicosis, is where the thyroid gland produces too much of the thyroid hormones T4, T3, or both.

What causes hyperthyroidism?

A variety of conditions can cause hyperthyroidism. Graves' disease, an autoimmune disorder, is the most common cause of hyperthyroidism. It causes antibodies to stimulate the thyroid to secrete too much hormone. Graves' disease occurs more often in women than in men. It tends to run in families, which suggests a genetic link. You should tell your doctor if your relatives have had the condition.

Other causes of hyperthyroidism include:

- excess iodine, a key ingredient in T4 and T3
- thyroiditis, or inflammation of the thyroid, which causes T4 and T3 to leak out of the gland
- tumours of the ovaries or testes
- benign tumours of the thyroid or pituitary gland
- large amounts of tetraiodothyronine taken through dietary supplements or medication

What are the symptoms of hyperthyroidism?

High amounts of T4, T3, or both can cause an excessively high metabolic rate. This is called a hypermetabolic state. When in a hypermetabolic state, you may experience a rapid heart rate, elevated blood pressure, and hand tremors. You may also sweat a lot and develop a low tolerance for heat. Hyperthyroidism can cause more frequent bowel movements, weight loss, and, in women, irregular menstrual cycles.

Other symptoms of hyperthyroidism include:

- increased appetite
- Nervousness
- goiter
- restlessness
- inability to concentrate
- weakness
- irregular heartbeat
- difficulty sleeping
- fine, brittle hair
- itching
- hair loss
- nausea and vomiting
- breast development in men

The following symptoms require immediate medical attention:

- dizziness
- shortness of breath
- loss of consciousness
- fast, irregular heart rate

Hyperthyroidism can also cause atrial fibrillation, a dangerous arrhythmia that can lead to strokes, as well as congestive heart failure.

How to diagnose hyperthyroidism?

Your first step in diagnosis is to get a complete medical history and physical exam. So, the diagnosis of the two types of thyroid issues are similar and can reveal these common signs of hyperthyroidism:

- weight loss
- rapid pulse
- elevated blood pressure
- protruding eyes
- enlarged thyroid gland

Other tests may be performed to further evaluate your diagnosis. These include:

Cholesterol test

Your doctor may need to check your cholesterol levels. Low cholesterol can be a sign of an elevated metabolic rate, in which your body is burning through cholesterol quickly.

T4, free T4, T3

These tests measure how much thyroid hormone (T4 and T3) is in your blood.

Thyroid stimulating hormone level test

Thyroid stimulating hormone (TSH) is a pituitary gland hormone that stimulates the thyroid gland to produce hormones. When thyroid hormone levels are normal or high, your TSH should be lower. An abnormally low TSH can be the first sign of hyperthyroidism.

Triglyceride test

Your triglyceride level may also be tested. Similar to low cholesterol, low triglycerides can be a sign of an elevated metabolic rate.

Thyroid scan and uptake

This allows your doctor to see if your thyroid is overactive. In particular, it can reveal whether the entire thyroid or just a single area of the gland is causing the overactivity.

Ultrasound

Ultrasounds can measure the size of the entire thyroid gland, as well as any masses within it. Doctors can also use ultrasounds to determine if a mass is solid or cystic.

CT or MRI scans

A CT or MRI can show if a pituitary tumour is present that's causing the condition.

How to treat hyperthyroidism?

Medication

Antithyroid medications, such as methimazole (Tapazole), stop the thyroid from making hormones. They are a common treatment.

Radioactive iodine

Radioactive iodine is given to over 70 percent of U.S. adults with hyperthyroidism, according to the American Thyroid Association. It effectively destroys the cells that produce hormones.

Common side effects include dry mouth, dry eyes, sore throat, and changes in taste. Precautions may need to be taken for a short time after treatment to prevent radiation spread to others.

Surgery

A section or all of your thyroid gland may be surgically removed. You will then have to take thyroid hormone supplements to prevent hypothyroidism, which occurs when you have an underactive thyroid that secretes too little hormone. Also, beta-blockers such as propranolol can help control your rapid pulse, sweating, anxiety, and high blood pressure. Most people respond well to this treatment.

What you can do to improve symptoms

Eating a proper diet, with a focus on calcium and sodium, is important, especially in preventing hyperthyroidism. Work with your doctor to create healthy guidelines for your diet, nutritional supplements, and exercise.

Hyperthyroidism can also cause your bones to become weak and thin, which can lead to osteoporosis. Taking vitamin D and calcium supplements during and after treatment can help strengthen your bones. Your doctor can tell you how much vitamin D and calcium to take each day.

Conclusion

Your doctor may refer you to an endocrinologist, who specializes in treating bodily hormone systems. Stress or infections can cause a thyroid storm. Thyroid storm happens when a large amount of thyroid hormone is released and it results in a sudden worsening of symptoms. Treatment is important to prevent thyroid storm, thyrotoxicosis, and other complications.

The long-term outlook for hyperthyroidism depends on its cause. Some causes can go away without treatment. Others, like Graves' disease, get worse over time without treatment. The complications of Graves' disease can be life-threatening and affect your long-term quality of life. Early diagnosis and treatment of symptoms improve the long-term outlook.

It's important to note that your body naturally goes

through changes as you get older and if you feel your symptoms are worsening with age, talk to your doctor to see if a thyroid problem may be affecting you.

Keep a log of the symptoms you may have and present them to your doctor and a diagnosis can be made and symptoms can be managed.

If you are someone who is trying to lose weight, once your medication is at the right dosage then there should not be any issues once you are living a balanced diet, exercising regularly and you are in a caloric deficit. Exercise can really help mood, joints and overall cardiac health. It is crucial that some sort of daily movement occurs.

Chapter 10 - Your cycle leaves clues

The final chapter in the book talks about some of the most common issues that women can face during their lifetime. If you track your cycle then you can see what is "normal" for you. Some of these symptoms are providing you feedback with what could be going elsewhere in your life or your body. Nothing happens for no reason.

Period Pain

This section is about normal period pain - not the severe pain that may come alongside Endometriosis or PCOS.

It's important to note that it's more common than you realise to feel discomfort around your abdomen, lower back and thighs when you are menstruating. At present it's unknown as to why some women will suffer more than others so more research is needed in this area to fully understand the reasons. But some factors that are associated with more intense pain include:

- having a heavy blood flow
- having your first child
- being under the age of 20, or just starting your period
- other factors include growths in your womb, endometriosis (abnormal uterine tissue growth), and use of birth control.

One of the main causes of period pain is a hormone called prostaglandin that triggers muscle contractions in your uterus that expel the lining.

These contractions can cause pain and inflammation. The level of prostaglandin rises right before menstruation begins. Too many prostaglandins can cause the pain and the main treatment is to reduce these prostaglandins.

Treatments for Period Pain

Over the counter (OTC) medications

Over the counter medications such as Ibuprofen (Advil or Nurofen) help lower your body's production of prostaglandin which ultimately relieves period pain. It's important to be aware that relying on Ibuprofen is only a short-term solution and that once you find a more natural treatment you will probably find that you will not need these medications as often or at all.

Applying heat

Applying heat to your abdomen and lower back may relieve pain. A 2012 study focused on 147 women 18 to 30 years old who had regular menstrual cycles found that a heat patch at 104°F (40°C) was as effective as ibuprofen. You can use a hot water bottle, a heating pad or if you don't have either of those you can also use a hot towel.

Massages

One 2010 study looked at 23 women with period pain caused by Endometriosis. The researchers found that massages significantly reduced pain immediately afterwards.

The research would indicate that 20 minutes of massage therapy can help reduce menstrual pain. If you add in some essential oils this has shown to have additional benefits.

A 2012 study divided 48 women experiencing menstrual pain into two groups: One group received a cream containing essential oils, while the other received a cream containing a synthetic fragrance.

The group who used essential oils experienced a significant reduction in amount and duration of pain.

Having an orgasm

While there are no clinical studies on the direct effect of orgasms on menstrual cramps, science suggests it may help.

A study carried out in 1985 by Dr. Beth Whipple was the first to find that vaginal self-stimulation doubled women's tolerance for pain.

Reducing certain foods

Reducing doesn't mean to take out or restrict (unless you have an intolerance or trying a FODMAP diet). Some foods can cause bloating and water retention. It is important to note that every woman will be different when it comes to what foods may cause this, so it could be an idea to keep a log or a diary of the types of the foods that are causing the bloating and reduce these from there.
Some foods that can have this impact on people

are:

- fatty foods
- alcohol
- carbonated beverages
- chewing gum
- caffeine
- salty foods

Reducing or cutting out these foods (depending on symptoms) can help alleviate cramps and decrease tension.

Adding herbs to your diet

Some experts believe that some herbal remedies contain anti-inflammatory and antispasmodic compounds that can reduce the muscle contractions and swelling associated with menstrual pain.

Some of these herbs include:

- *Chamomile tea* - A 2012 review of studies reports chamomile tea increases urinary levels of glycine, which helps relieve muscle spasms. Glycine also acts as a nerve relaxant. Sipping two cups of tea per day a week before your period may be of benefit.
- *Ginger* - One study of university students found that 250 mg of ginger powder four times a day for three days helped with pain relief. It also concluded ginger was as effective as ibuprofen. Start by grating a small piece of ginger into hot water for a warm cramp-relieving drink.

- *Dill* - A 2014 study concluded 1,000 mg dill was as effective for easing menstrual cramps as mefenamic acid, an OTC drug for menstrual pain. Try 1,000 mg of dill for five days, starting two days before your cycle.
- *Curcumin* (a natural chemical in turmeric) - may help with symptoms of premenstrual syndrome (PMS). One 2015 study looked at 70 women who took two capsules of curcumin for seven days before their period and three days after. Participants reported significant reduction in PMS.

Please do not try these together and please talk to your doctor before you take them.

Identify and treat histamine intolerance

Histamine intolerance is another cause of period pain. It is caused by having too much of the inflammatory compound histamine. This could have an impact on headaches, anxiety, insomnia, brain fog and hives to name a few symptoms. It can also worsen period problems because it increases both inflammation and estrogen. PMS and period pain are two of the most common symptoms with histamine intolerance.

You will need to always make sure you're buying herbs and supplements from a reputable source as they aren't regulated. While most of these herbal remedies are great some may have some side effects, check with your doctor before trying them as some can have unintended side effects with certain medications.

What about Nutrition and Exercise?

Exercise

The idea of doing any exercise around your time of the month may not appeal to you in any way. But guess what? Exercise releases Endorphins (the happy hormone) which can help to improve overall mood.

Research suggests exercise is effective at reducing menstrual pain to the extent it may also eliminate or reduce the need for pain-relief medication. Moderate activity such as walking can be beneficial during your period in place of more strenuous activity.

Yoga is also a great form of movement around this time of the month as it is a gentle form of exercise that also releases endorphins and helps prevent or reduce menstrual symptoms.

Reducing running and HIIT (high intensity exercise) can also aid managing your period pain. This is a time to be sound to yourself so please be patient with you.

Nutrition and Supplementation around this time

A diet that has minimally processed foods around this time will suit you a lot more. So aim to increase the likes of the foods below:

- Papaya is rich in vitamins.

- Brown rice contains vitamin B-6, which may reduce bloating (think wholegrain)
- Walnuts, almonds, and pumpkin seeds are rich in manganese, which eases cramps.
- Olive oil and broccoli contain vitamin E.
- Chicken, fish, and leafy green vegetables contain iron, which is lost during menstruation.
- Flaxseed contains omega-3s with antioxidant properties, which reduce swelling and inflammation.
- *Water* - It sounds odd, but drinking water keeps your body from retaining water and helps to avoid painful bloating during menstruation. Warm or hot water is usually better for cramps, as hot liquids increase blood flow to your skin and may relax cramped muscles
- *Magnesium* - gold standard for period pain. It reduces the prostaglandins and relaxes the uterus. The dose would be 100mg to 300mg of magnesium glycinate per day. Start on the lower dose first.
- *Zinc* - prevents period pain by inhibiting prostaglandins and inflammation. Try 20-50mg as a daily dose.

Magnesium and Zinc are a great place to start alongside managing your nutrition as best you can. Make sure if you are getting herbal remedies that they do not interact with your current medications and to get the ok from the doctor before you take them.

Early Periods

The next section we are going to look at early periods. There is generally a reason for your cycle appearing either early or late. So please make sure you know what's normal for you. Nothing happens for no reason.

Just a quick recap before we go any further, everyone's menstrual cycle is different. Your cycle starts on the first day of your current period and ends on the first day of your next period.

A typical cycle lasts anywhere from 25-39 days, so the number of days spent bleeding varies from person to person. Most people bleed for two to seven days. (check out the chapter on the menstrual cycle for more detail)

If your cycle is frequently shorter than 24 days — leading you to bleed earlier than you normally do — it could be a sign of something underlying.

There are many possible causes of irregular periods. Sometimes they may just be normal for you.

Common causes include:

- Puberty – your periods might be irregular for the first year or two
- The start of the menopause (usually between the ages of 45 and 55)
- Early pregnancy – take a pregnancy test to rule this out

- Some types of hormonal contraception – such as the contraceptive pill or intrauterine system (IUS)
- Extreme weight loss or weight gain, excessive exercise or stress
- Medical conditions – such as polycystic ovary syndrome (PCOS)
- Thyroid
- Low progesterone

The topic of progesterone has been spoken about in the menstrual cycle chapter but here is a quick recap.

Progesterone is important during childbearing years. If you don't have enough progesterone, you may have trouble getting or staying pregnant.

Low progesterone may cause abnormal uterine bleeding in women who aren't pregnant. Irregular or absent periods may indicate poorly functioning ovaries and low progesterone.

Symptoms of low progesterone in women who aren't pregnant include:

- headaches or migraines
- mood changes, including anxiety or depression
- irregularity in menstrual cycle

Think of progesterone as your calming hormone and estrogen as your hormone that gets you horny and passion comes from. Your Ying to your yang.

Without progesterone to complement it, estrogen may become the dominant hormone. This may cause symptoms including:

- weight gain
- decreased sex drive, mood swings, and depression
- PMS, irregular menstrual cycle, heavy bleeding
- breast tenderness, fibrocystic breasts
- fibroids
- gallbladder problems

The best way to get your progesterone levels checked is to chat with your doctor and get a blood test. The best day to get a test is the middle of your luteal phase. The day this occurs will differ for each individual so it is imperative that you know the duration of your cycle through tracking and even checking your waking temperature. The mid luteal day is approximately seven days after ovulation and seven days before your next expected period.

If tested at the right time (after ovulation) then the results should be at least 3 ng/ml (9.5nmol/L). If it is below that then you did not ovulate or you took the test at the wrong time. When asking your doctor for guidance, knowing when you are ovulating and when the middle of your cycle will help to get a diagnosis quicker. A decent progesterone level is 10ng/ml (30nmol/L) and it may be much higher. The higher the better!

Charting your waking temperature can also help. If you consistently see a rise in temperature and a luteal phase of at least 11 days then you may know you have made enough progesterone.

Tips for management

- Use a period app. Period tracking apps allow you to log your day-to-day symptoms. Over time, you may notice a pattern in your flow. You can also share your logs with your doctor at your next appointment.
- Stay prepared. Keep a few panty liners, pads, or tampons in your bag or at work so you aren't caught off guard. For added protection, consider investing in a set of period underwear. Running out?
- Get some sleep.
- Eat a balanced diet.
- Don't train too hard and take rest days.
- Manage your stress.
- Maintain a healthy weight. Obesity can interfere with your reproductive hormones.
- See a doctor - if you're in severe pain or discomfort, you should see your doctor.

If you aren't experiencing any severe symptoms, you may be able to regulate things at home. Consider tracking your periods for the next two to three months to see how your timing, flow, and other symptoms compare.

If things aren't levelling out, talk to your doctor. They can use this information to evaluate your cycle and advise you on any next steps.

Spotting

Spotting is defined as light vaginal bleeding that happens outside of your regular periods. Typically, spotting involves small amounts of blood. It's typically not a sign of something serious but it is definitely something that should not be ignored and the best advice is talk to your doctor if it occurs.

Your doctor can help you understand why spotting is happening. There are steps you can take on your own to help to reduce it too, but we need to understand why the spotting is happening.

<u>Why is the spotting happening?</u>

When you go to the doctor a number of questions will be asked. The questions will look back through your menstrual history including the length and type of bleeding that normally occurs.

After gathering this information on your general health your doctor may give you a physical exam and additional tests may be ordered. Some of these may tests include:

- blood test
- Pap test
- ultrasound
- hysteroscopy
- MRI scan
- CT scan
- endometrial biopsy

There are two main types of spotting, Ovulation

Spotting and Premenstrual Spotting.

Ovulation spotting generally occurs when your estrogen dips a little just before your LH surge and egg release and the colour is typically bright red when this happens.

While premenstrual spotting is a darker colour and it can mean you do not have enough progesterone to hold your uterine lining.

What's causing the spotting and what can be done?

Spotting can be a sign of a number of conditions. Some can be treated by your doctor, while others can be addressed with self-care. Self-care is something that we can all do a bit better on.

Some of the conditions include:

Pregnancy

When a fertilized egg is implanted in your uterine lining, implantation bleeding can occur. If you have missed an expected period and think you might be pregnant, consider taking a home pregnancy test. If you believe you're pregnant, see an OB-GYN to confirm your test results and talk about next steps.

Thyroid condition

Hormones produced by your thyroid help control your menstrual cycle. Too much or too little thyroid hormone can make your periods very light, heavy, or irregular. These conditions are known as hyperthyroidism and hypothyroidism.

Hyperthyroidism is commonly treated with antithyroid medications or beta-blockers. Surgery to remove all or some of the thyroid might be recommended. Hypothyroidism is commonly treated with man-made forms of the hormone that your thyroid should be making.

Please see the previous chapter for more information on issues with Thyroid).

Medication

Some medications can cause spotting as a side effect. Examples include:
- anticoagulants
- corticosteroids
- tricyclic antidepressants
- phenothiazines

If you take any of these prescription medications and experience spotting, speak with your doctor.

Stress

A 2005 study in young women showed a relationship between high stress and menstrual irregularities.

You can manage and relieve stress by:

- staying physically active

- eating a healthy diet
- getting enough sleep
- practicing relaxation techniques, such as meditation, yoga, and massage

If these self-care methods aren't effective for you, consider asking your doctor for their suggestions on stress relief and management.

Weight Management

According to a 2017 study, weight management and changes in body weight can affect the regulation of your menstrual cycle and cause spotting.

You can limit these effects by maintaining a consistent weight. Work with a Nutritionist or a Coach who can help you with this.

Spotting and contraceptives

If you start, stop, skip, or change oral birth control, you might experience some spotting.

Changing birth control can change your estrogen level. Since estrogen helps keep your uterine lining in place, spotting might occur as your body tries to adjust when estrogen levels are changed.

According to a 2016 study, spotting can also be caused by other forms of birth control, including:

- *Implant* - Spotting is common with the etonogestrel implant.

- *Injectable* - Spotting is common with depot medroxyprogesterone acetate (DMPA), an injectable form of progestin only contraception.
- *IUD* - As a foreign body in your uterus, a hormonal or copper intrauterine device (IUD) can cause spotting.

Other factors that may cause spotting include STIs, Medications, ovarian cysts and cancer.

<u>When to go to your doctor?</u>

Although spotting is not uncommon, consult with your doctor or OB-GYN if any of the following occur:

- it happens more than a couple of times
- there's no obvious explanation
- you're pregnant
- it occurs after menopause
- it increases to heavy bleeding
- you experience pain, fatigue, or dizziness in addition to spotting

There are many potential causes for spotting. Some need professional medical treatment, while others you can handle with self-care. Either way, it's important to see your doctor to diagnose the underlying cause. Nothing happens for no reason so it is important to get to the root cause of the issue.

Your body is providing you with feedback so it's up to you to make sure you understand your body and listen to it. This could lead to freedom.

Ovarian cysts

The next section is ovarian cysts. Your ovaries always have "cysts" or fluid filled sacs. Many women will develop at least one cyst during their lifetime. In most cases, cysts are painful and cause no symptoms.

<u>There are a number of types of ovarian cysts</u>

There are various types of ovarian cysts, such as dermoid cysts and endometrioma cysts. However, functional cysts are the most common type.

Dermoid cysts are sac-like growths on the ovaries that can contain hair, fat, and other tissue cystadenomas: noncancerous growths that can develop on the outer surface of the ovaries endometriomas: tissues that normally grow inside the uterus can develop outside the uterus and attach to the ovaries, resulting in a cyst.

Some women develop a condition called polycystic ovary syndrome. This condition means the ovaries contain a large number of small cysts. It can cause the ovaries to enlarge. If left untreated, polycystic ovaries can cause infertility. Please check out the PCOS chapter for more detail on this.

<u>Treatment for an ovarian cyst</u>

Your doctor may recommend treatment to shrink or remove the cyst if it doesn't go away on its own or if it grows larger.

Some of the other treatments may include:

Birth control pills

If you have recurrent ovarian cysts, your doctor can prescribe oral contraceptives to stop ovulation and prevent the development of new cysts. Oral contraceptives can also reduce your risk of ovarian cancer. The risk of ovarian cancer is higher in postmenopausal women.

Laparoscopy

If your cyst is small and results from an imaging test to rule out cancer, your doctor can perform a laparoscopy to surgically remove the cyst. The procedure involves your doctor making a tiny incision near your navel and then inserting a small instrument into your abdomen to remove the cyst.

Laparotomy

If you have a large cyst, your doctor can surgically remove the cyst through a large incision in your abdomen. They'll conduct an immediate biopsy, and if they determine that the cyst is cancerous, they may perform a hysterectomy to remove your ovaries and uterus.

Some research has shown that supplementation of Iodine (down regulates and stabilises estrogen receptors) and Selenium (promotes healthy ovulation and aids in the formation of the formation of the corpus luteum) but more research is needed on this to confirm its validity. Please check with your doctor before taking this approach.

What can be done for Ovarian cyst prevention?

Ovarian cysts can't be prevented. However, routine gynecologic examinations can detect ovarian cysts early. It's important to visit your doctor and receive a correct diagnosis.

If left untreated, some cysts can decrease fertility. This is common with endometriosis and polycystic ovary syndrome. To improve fertility, your doctor can remove or shrink the cyst. Functional cysts, cystadenomas, and dermoid cysts do not affect fertility.

The outlook for premenopausal women with ovarian cysts is good. Most cysts disappear within a few months. However, recurrent ovarian cysts can occur in premenopausal women and women with hormone imbalances. Check with your doctor on this.

Heavy periods

Heavy menstrual bleeding can affect up to 1 in 4 women so it is important to know what is normal for you and your cycle. I will always revert back at the importance of tracking your cycle and how it provides you with feedback on what happens at the various stages of your cycle.

If something then changes from this "norm" for you then you know something is up. Remember nothing happens for no reason.

So, let's look at what is normal for the flow of your

cycle. Your menstrual fluid should be bright red, no clots and most liquid. Your period should not be painful (please refer back to the section of how to manage painful periods).

The duration and severity of menstrual bleeding varies from woman to woman. If your menstrual period is excessively heavy, prolonged, or irregular, it's known as menorrhagia.

Symptoms of menorrhagia include

- a menstrual period that lasts longer than seven days
- bleeding so heavy that you must change your tampon or pad more than once per hour

You should see your doctor if you have excessively heavy or prolonged menstrual periods that interfere with your daily life. If you are losing more than 80mL then this is not menorrhagia it is called menstrual flooding and can sometimes happen during perimenopause.

Excessive bleeding can cause anaemia, or iron deficiency. It may also signal an underlying medical condition. In most cases, your doctor can successfully treat abnormal periods.

What are the main causes of heavy or irregular menstrual periods?

Heavy or irregular periods can be due to a variety of factors, including:

Medications

Some anti-inflammatory drugs, anticoagulants, or hormone medications can affect menstrual bleeding. Heavy bleeding can be a side effect of intrauterine devices (IUDs) used for birth control. It's important to know that you have options when it comes to the type of birth control you use (please check the chapter on birth control for more information).

Hormone imbalances

The hormones estrogen and progesterone regulate the build-up of the lining of the uterus. An excess of these hormones can cause heavy bleeding.

Hormone imbalances are most common among girls who began menstruating in the past year and a half. They're also common in women who are getting close to menopause. It is important to go to a doctor if you feel it may be Endometriosis or PCOS, and look at all options that are available.

Endometriosis

Endometriosis is another condition that can result in irregular periods. This is a condition in which tissue that lines the inside of the uterus begins to grow elsewhere inside the body. This can cause heavy bleeding, as well as pain (see chapter on Endometriosis)

Inherited blood disorder
Heavy menstrual bleeding can be due to some

inherited blood disorders that affect clotting. Willebrand disease or haemophilia but there are other several ones. Your doctor can rule out a blood disorder through a simple blood screening. If something does appear, knowing that you have options will really help and your doctor may refer you to a specialist or a haematologist.

Thyroid Disease

Underactive thyroid or hypothyroidism is a common cause of heavy menstrual bleeding. But it's important to mention this to the doctor when discussing options and not all doctors will consider this. Please revert back to the chapter on Thyroid for more information.

There are several mechanisms by which an underactive thyroid can make periods heavier:

- Without sufficient thyroid hormone, your ovaries may not be able to make enough of the flow-decreasing hormone progesterone.
- Without sufficient thyroid hormone, you may not make enough of the coagulation factors you need to prevent heavy bleeding.
- Without sufficient thyroid hormone, you make less of the estrogen-binding protein SHBG and so are exposed to more estrogen.
- "Unopposed estrogen," which means a hormone imbalance of too much estrogen and not enough progesterone

If your healthcare provider discovers that you have an underactive thyroid, then your best treatment for heavy periods may be to take thyroid hormone.

Other medical reasons for heavy periods include benign growths or cancers, liver disease, pelvic infection, miscarriage, uterine polyps, fibroids, anovulation (lack of ovulation), Adenomyosis and Ectopic pregnancy.

Seek immediate medical attention if you bleed heavily during pregnancy. It can be a sign that the fertilized egg is implanted in the fallopian tube rather than the uterus, which is called an ectopic pregnancy. It can also indicate a miscarriage.

Your doctor will be able to help you determine what's causing any bleeding during pregnancy.

What are the symptoms of heavy or irregular periods?

The length of the menstrual cycle and amount of blood flow is unique to each woman. Please track your cycle. I cannot say this enough.

Blood flow averages about four or five days, with a blood loss of about 40 cc (3 tablespoons). It's important to remember that these are just averages. Your "normal" may fall outside of these ranges. A blood loss of 80 cc (5 tablespoons) or more is considered an abnormally heavy flow.

Signs that your menstrual flow may be abnormally heavy include:

- soaking through more than one tampon or sanitary pad in an hour for several hours at a time
- waking up during the night because you need to change protection
- passing large blood clots in your menstrual flow
- experiencing a menstrual flow that lasts more than a week

Please make sure that you talk to your doctor to make sure all is ok.

While every woman's cycle is different, irregularities such as bleeding mid-cycle or bleeding after intercourse are abnormal symptoms.

<u>When should you seek medical care?</u>

You should see your gynaecologist regularly for a check-up. However, make an appointment right away if you have bleeding or spotting in the following circumstances:

- between periods
- after sex
- while pregnant
- after menopause

Other indicators that you should contact your doctor include the following:

- if your periods consistently last for more than a week

- if you require more than one tampon or sanitary pad in an hour, for several hours in a row
- severe pain
- fever
- abnormal discharge or odour
- unexplained weight gain or loss
- unusual hair growth
- new acne
- nipple discharge

Keep track of your menstrual cycles, including how long your blood flow lasts, and how many tampons or sanitary pads you use during each cycle. This information will be helpful at your gynaecological appointment.

Avoid products that contain aspirin because they may increase bleeding.

What are the treatment options for heavy or irregular menstrual periods?

Everyone is different and the type of treatment. You should discuss benefits and risks of the different options with your doctor, including any impact on future fertility from some treatments.
The type of treatment will depend on a number of things including:

- your overall health
- the reason for your menstrual abnormalities
- your reproductive history and future plans

- Your doctor will also need to address any underlying medical conditions, such as thyroid dysfunction.

Treatments may include the following.

Intrauterine system (IUS)

The IUS, or levonorgestrel-releasing intrauterine system, is a small plastic device inserted into your womb by a doctor or nurse. It slowly releases a hormone called progestogen.

It prevents the lining of your womb growing quickly and is also a contraceptive. An IUS doesn't affect your chances of getting pregnant after you stop using it.

Possible side effects of using an IUS include:

- irregular bleeding that may last more than 6 months
- breast tenderness
- acne
- stopped or missed periods
- An IUS is often the preferred first treatment for women with heavy menstrual bleeding, but it can take at least 6 periods for you to start seeing the benefits.

Tranexamic acid

You may be prescribed tranexamic acid tablets if an IUS is unsuitable or you're waiting for further tests or another treatment.

The tablets work by helping the blood in your womb to clot. Tranexamic acid tablets are usually taken 3 times a day for a maximum of 4 days. You start taking the tablets as soon as your period starts.

Tranexamic acid tablets are not a form of contraception and won't affect your chances of becoming pregnant. If necessary, tranexamic acid can be combined with a non-steroidal anti-inflammatory drug (NSAID).

Possible side effects of tranexamic acid include:

- diarrhoea
- feeling sick
- being sick

Non-steroidal anti-inflammatory drugs (NSAIDs)

NSAIDs can also be used to treat heavy periods if an IUS isn't appropriate, or if you're waiting for further tests or a different treatment.

They're taken in tablet form from the start of or just before your period, until heavy bleeding has stopped. NSAIDs used for treating heavy menstrual bleeding include:

- ibuprofen
- mefenamic acid
- naproxen
- Mefenamic acid and naproxen are only available on prescription.

NSAIDs work by reducing your body's production of a hormone-like substance called prostaglandin, which is linked to heavy periods. NSAIDs can also help relieve period pain. They're not a form of contraceptive.

You can keep taking NSAIDs for as long as you need to if they're making your bleeding less heavy and not causing significant side effects.

Make sure you do not take more than the recommended daily dose listed on the packet.

Combined oral contraceptive pill

The combined contraceptive pill can be used to treat heavy periods. It contains the hormones estrogen and progestogen.

The benefit of using combined oral contraceptives as a treatment for heavy periods is they offer a more readily reversible form of contraception than the IUS.

They also have the benefit of regulating your menstrual cycle and reducing period pain.

The pill works by preventing your ovaries releasing an egg each month. As long as you're taking it correctly, it should prevent pregnancy.
Common side effects of the combined oral contraceptive pill include:

- mood changes
- feeling sick (nausea)
- headaches
- breast tenderness

- Read more about the combined pill.

Cyclical progestogens

If other treatments have not helped, you may be offered a type of medicine called cyclical progestogen.

It's taken in tablet form for part of your menstrual cycle. Your doctor will advise you how to take it. It's not an effective form of contraception and can have unpleasant side effects, including:

- breast tenderness
- bleeding between your periods

Other options include Endometrial ablation, Uterine artery embolisation (UAE), Myomectomy or removal of the womb (hysterectomy). Please note there are other options available. It is so important that you know all of your options and talk to your doctor about these. You have the right to look at the best option for you so please do not feel under pressure to pick one.

What can you do with your diet and exercise?

Sometimes, food is the best medicine. Getting more iron in your diet can help reduce heavy bleeding and prevent anaemia caused by blood loss. Try eating iron-rich foods like meat, seafood, beans, nuts, seeds and leafy green vegetables.
If you are deficient or think you may be deficient in something please get blood tests done through companies like LetsGetChecked or chat with your

GP.

Eating foods with lots of vitamin C like oranges, bell peppers and broccoli can help your body absorb the extra iron in your diet. Also, do your best to reduce foods with processed sugar, trans-fats and starchy carbs. These foods can make menorrhagia symptoms worse.

Exercise will help to reduce inflammation and will promote the healthy removel of estrogen through perspiration.

Supplements

Iron

There's some evidence that suggests a lack of iron might contribute to heavy periods. If eating an iron-rich diet hasn't improved your levels, supplementation may help. If you are deficient or you think you are deficient you need to ask your doctor to get a scrum ferritin test. Your doctor should provide you with your options from here.

Turmeric

Including turmeric in your daily diet during periods could very well have beneficial effects for women who are going through heavy periods. Since turmeric has anti-inflammatory properties, it can help effectively during heavy flow.

Other supplements that have shown some

promising research include calcium-d-glucarate, vitamin c and micronized progesterone.

If you are having heavy periods, it is important to talk to your doctor and look at your full list of options. If you are over 40 the options may be different so please be aware of this.

Light periods

It is essential that you understand what is "normal" for your body and for your period. Remember every woman is different.

Your period can be heavy but it can also be light and it is important to know why this occurs. A period comes when the lining of your uterus sheds through your cervix and vagina, generally on a monthly basis. A light period is a sign of lower-than-average estrogen.

Some of the common symptoms of a light period that you may be concerned about include:

- you bleed for fewer than two days
- your bleeding is very light, like spotting
- you miss one or more regular-flow periods
- you experience more frequent light periods than the typical 21- to 35-day cycle

Remember that you may experience an unusual period for no particular reason, but you should still let your doctor know. They can help determine any underlying causes that may be affecting your menstrual cycle and vaginal bleeding.

Some of the common causes of a light period include:

Age

Your period can vary in length and flow if you are in your teenage years. On the flip side, if you are in menopause, you may experience irregular periods that are light in flow. These occurrences are the result of hormonal imbalances.

Weight and diet

Body weight and body fat percentage can affect your period. Being extremely underweight can cause your period to become irregular because your hormones are not working normally. Additionally, losing or gaining an extreme amount of weight can cause irregularities with your period.

Pregnancy

If you are pregnant, it is unlikely that you will have a period. You may notice some spotting and think it's your period, but it may actually be implantation bleeding. This can occur when a fertilized egg attaches to the lining of the uterus. Implantation bleeding usually lasts for two days or less.

Breast-feeding

If you are breast-feeding, your periods may not come back immediately after you give birth. The milk production hormone prevents ovulation and delays your period from returning. You may get your period months after giving birth if you are breast-feeding, while others may get it back in a quicker space of time.

Birth control

Hormonal birth control may be the cause of a light period (please check the chapter on birth control for more detail on each type). Some birth control methods prevent an egg from releasing in your body. These methods come in various forms, including:

- pill
- patch
- ring
- Shot

When your body doesn't release an egg, your uterus doesn't create a thick lining. This can result in lighter periods or skipped periods altogether. You may also experience irregular periods if you have started or stopped taking birth control recently. If you are worried in any way, please talk to your doctor about this.

Stress

If you're stressed, your brain can alter the menstrual cycle hormones. Not many people realise how the impact of stress can have on hormones and you may experience skipped or lighter periods because of it. Once a stressful event passes, your periods should return to normal.

Overexercising

Women who exercise frequently may experience changes to their period. Athletes can be under stress, have low body weight, and use a lot of body energy. This can result in altered periods.

The amount of exercise someone can tolerate is very personal but if you feel things are changing with your cycle and exercise is playing a factor, please talk to your doctor to know the next step. It can be altered for you based on the person. Please refer to the chapter on Hypothalamic Amenorrhea if you have lost your cycle completely.

Eating disorders

Anorexia nervosa and bulimia are types of eating disorders that may cause irregular periods. Eating disorders can lead to low body weight, which can alter hormones that regulate your period.

Polycystic ovary syndrome (PCOS)

If you're experiencing irregular periods or have stopped menstruating, it could be the result of PCOS. This causes a hormonal change in your body where your eggs stop maturing. Please check

Serious medical conditions can also be a factor. Unusual or irregular periods may be a sign of a more serious health condition. Discussing symptoms with your doctor may help you determine the cause of lighter than normal periods.

Treatment

Your light period may be caused by one of many factors. It may be a one-time occurrence. If your light periods persist or you experience any troubling symptoms, you may need further treatment.

Persistent and problematic light periods may be treated with changes to your lifestyle and medications. If the problem is persistent then you need to talk to your doctor and understand what options are available to you.

Uterine Fibroids

If your doctor has ordered a pelvic ultrasound to investigate the heavy bleeding or pain, they might discover a fibroid or fibroids. Many women have uterine fibroids sometime during their lives.

So, we need to look at what a fibroid is. Uterine fibroids are noncancerous growths of the uterus that often appear during childbearing years. Also called leiomyomas or myomas, uterine fibroids aren't associated with an increased risk of uterine cancer and almost never develop into cancer.

Fibroids range in size from seedlings, undetectable by the human eye, to bulky masses that can distort and enlarge the uterus. In extreme cases, multiple fibroids can expand the uterus so much that it reaches the rib cage and can add weight.

Symptoms

Many women who have fibroids don't have any symptoms. In women who have symptoms, the most common signs and symptoms of uterine fibroids include:

- Heavy menstrual bleeding
- Menstrual periods lasting more than a week
- Pelvic pressure or pain
- Frequent urination
- Difficulty emptying the bladder
- Constipation
- Backache or leg pains

Fibroids are generally classified by their location. There are a few main types of fibroids and they include Intramural fibroids (that grow within the muscular uterine wall), Submucosal fibroids (they bulge into the uterine cavity) and Subserosal fibroids (they project to the outside of the uterus).

It's unclear why fibroids develop, but several factors like Hormones, Family history and Pregnancy may play a role.

Risk factors include anything that may increase your exposure to estrogen. In one study there was a link with an increased risk of developing fibroids with the pill and taking it at a younger age. More research is needed. Alcohol consumption can also play a role in the development of fibroids due to its link to increasing estrogen.

For a proper diagnosis, you'll need to see a

gynaecologist to get a pelvic exam. You may also need other tests, which include an Ultrasound or a pelvic MRI.

How are fibroids treated?

Your doctor will develop a treatment plan based on your age, the size of your fibroids, and your overall health. You may receive a combination of treatments. It's important to note that fibroids are easier to prevent than they are to treat.

Unless the fibroid is large or goring inside your uterus it will not require medical attention. It's important to note that fibroids will reduce in size with menopause.

Some of the treatments that may be offered to help with fibroids include a Hysterectomy, Myomectomy, Uterine artery embolisation (UAE) or a Hysteroscopic resection of fibroids. Your doctor will be able to provide you with all of the various options. Surgery to remove your fibroids may be considered if your symptoms are particularly severe and medicine has been ineffective.

Hysterectomy

A hysterectomy is a surgical procedure to remove the womb. It's the most effective way of preventing fibroids coming back.

A hysterectomy may be recommended if you have large fibroids or severe bleeding and do not wish to have any more children. There are a number of different ways a hysterectomy can be carried out, including through the vagina or through a number of small cuts (incisions) in your tummy (abdomen).

Depending on the technique used, a hysterectomy can be carried out using a spinal or epidural anaesthetic, where the lower parts of the body are numbed. Sometimes a general anaesthetic may be used, where you'll be asleep during the procedure.

Side effects of a hysterectomy can include early menopause and a loss of libido (sex drive). This usually only occurs if the ovaries have been removed.

Myomectomy

A myomectomy is surgery to remove the fibroids from the wall of your womb. It may be considered as an alternative to a hysterectomy if you'd still like to have children.

But a myomectomy is not suitable for all types of fibroids. Your gynaecologist can tell you whether the procedure is suitable for you based on factors such as the size, number and position of your fibroids.

Depending on the size and position of your fibroids, a myomectomy may involve making either a number of small incisions in your tummy (keyhole surgery) or a single larger incision (open surgery).

Myomectomies are carried out under general anaesthetic and you'll usually need to stay in hospital for a few days afterwards. You'll be advised to rest for several weeks while you recover.

Myomectomies are usually an effective treatment for fibroids, although there's a chance the fibroids will grow back and further surgery will be needed.

Uterine artery embolisation (UAE)

Uterine artery embolisation (UAE) is an alternative procedure to a hysterectomy or myomectomy for treating fibroids. It may be recommended for women with large fibroids.

UAE is carried out by a radiologist. It involves blocking the blood vessels that supply the fibroids, causing them to shrink. During the procedure, a special solution is injected through a small tube (catheter), which is guided by X-ray through a blood vessel in your leg.

Although it's possible to have a successful pregnancy after having UAE, the overall effects of the procedure on fertility and pregnancy are uncertain.

It should therefore only be carried out after you have discussed the potential risks, benefits and uncertainties with your doctor.

Hysteroscopic morcellation of fibroids

Hysteroscopic morcellation of fibroids is a new procedure where a clinician who's received specialist training uses a hysteroscope and small surgical instruments to remove fibroids.

The hysteroscope is inserted into the womb through the cervix and a specially designed instrument called a morcellator is used to cut away and remove the fibroid tissue.

The procedure is carried out under a general or spinal anaesthetic. You'll usually be able to go home on the same day.

The main benefit of hysteroscopic morcellation compared with hysteroscopic resection is that the hysteroscope is only inserted once, rather than a number of times, reducing the risk of injury to the womb.

But because hysteroscopic morcellation is a new technique, evidence about its overall safety and long-term effectiveness is limited so it is important to talk with your doctor and specialist.

What about dietary and lifestyle changes?

It is important to note that natural treatment cannot substantially shrink fibroids, but it can further prevent further growth.

There are a number of changes you can make that might help reduce your risk for fibroids.

Follow a Mediterranean diet

Add plenty of fresh and cooked green vegetables, fresh fruit, legumes, and fish to your plate. A Mediterranean diet is one way to do this. Research shows that eating these foods regularly may help lower your risk for fibroids. On the other hand, eating an abundance of beef, ham, lamb, and other red meat may raise your risk.

Cut back on alcohol

Drinking any type of alcohol may increase your risk for fibroids. This can happen because alcohol raises the level of hormones (estrogen) needed for fibroids to grow. Alcohol may also trigger inflammation.

One study found that women who drank one or more beers a day increased their risk by more than 50 percent. Avoid or limit alcohol to help reduce your risk.

Maintaining a healthy weight

Obesity and excess weight increase the risk for fibroids. Fat cells make more estrogen, so losing weight may help prevent or slow the growth of fibroids.

Avoiding hormone-disrupting chemicals

Natural and synthetic chemicals can throw off your endocrine balance, raising estrogen levels. These chemicals can include the likes of fertilizers and pesticides etc.

Lower blood pressure

Research shows that a high number of women with severe fibroids also have high blood pressure. More research is needed to find out if there's a link.

Get enough vitamin D

Vitamin D may help reduce your risk of fibroids by almost 32 percent. Your body makes this "sunshine vitamin" naturally when your skin's exposed to sunlight. If you have darker skin or live-in cooler climates, you're more likely to be deficient.

Maintaining good gut health

Fibre-rich foods aid weight loss and balance hormones. They also help to keep blood sugar levels steady. For these reasons, fibre may help prevent and slow the growth of fibroids. Think of filling up your plate with lots of vegetables. The importance of good digestion cannot be downplayed as the main way for estrogen to be excreted from the body is through going for a poo.

Eating a balanced diet and maintaining a healthy weight is important for your overall health. You may not be able to prevent fibroids, no matter what precautions you take. See your doctor if you think you may be at risk or if you experience any changes in your health.

If you have fibroids, your doctor will determine the best type of treatment. Healthy diet and lifestyle changes are the first step to treating fibroids and relieving symptoms.

Adenomyosis

Adenomyosis occurs when the tissue that normally lines the uterus (endometrial tissue) grows into the muscular wall of the uterus. The displaced tissue continues to act normally — thickening, breaking down and bleeding — during each menstrual cycle. An enlarged uterus and painful, heavy periods can result.

The displaced tissue continues to act normally — thickening, breaking down and bleeding — during each menstrual cycle. An enlarged uterus and painful, heavy periods can result.

It is a different kind of abnormal growth in your uterine wall. It's similar to uterine fibroids and until recently it was mistaken as that.

Doctors aren't sure what causes adenomyosis, but the disease usually resolves after menopause. For women who have severe discomfort from adenomyosis, hormonal treatments can help. Removal of the uterus (hysterectomy) cures adenomyosis

Symptoms of this condition can be mild to severe. Some women may not experience any at all. The most common symptoms include:

- prolonged menstrual cramps
- spotting between periods
- heavy menstrual bleeding

- longer menstrual cycles than normal
- blood clots during menstrual bleeding
- pain during sex
- tenderness in the abdominal area

In relation to getting a diagnosis, a complete medical evaluation can help to determine the best course of treatment. Your doctor will first want to perform a physical exam to determine if your uterus is swollen. Many women with adenomyosis will have a uterus that's double or triple the normal size. The best form of diagnosis is from a pelvic ultrasound or MRI.

What treatments are available?

Women with mild forms of this condition may not require medical treatment. Your doctor may recommend treatment options if your symptoms interfere with your daily activities.

Treatments aimed at reducing the symptoms of adenomyosis include the following:

Anti-inflammatory medications

An example is ibuprofen. These medications can help to reduce blood flow during your period while also relieving severe cramps. The Mayo Clinic recommends starting anti-inflammatory medication two to three days before the start of your period and continuing to take it during your period. You should not use these medications if you're pregnant.

Hormonal treatments

These include oral contraceptives (birth control pills), progestin-only contraceptives (oral, injection, or an intrauterine device), and GnRH-analogs such as Lupron (leuprolide). Hormonal treatments can help to control increased estrogen levels that may be contributing to your symptoms. Intrauterine devices, such as Mirena, can last up to five years.

Other treatments include Endometrial ablation, Uterine artery embolization and Hysterectomy.

In relation to diet and supplementation it will similar to that of what is recommended with those suffering from endometriosis:

- Reducing alcohol
- Maintaining lots of fibre in the diet
- Fruit is your friend
- Reducing processed foods
- Turmeric and Zinc for supplementation

Adenomyosis isn't necessarily harmful. However, the symptoms can negatively affect your lifestyle. Some people have excessive bleeding and pelvic pain that may prevent them from enjoying normal activities such as sexual intercourse.

Women with adenomyosis are at an increased risk of anaemia and the condition has also been linked with anxiety, depression, and irritability.

It's important to note that Adenomyosis isn't the same as Endometriosis.

If you are unsure if you have Endometriosis or Adenomyosis there are various treatment options in between these extremes. This is because of the differences in where the misplaced endometrial tissue is located.
Discuss your treatment options with your doctor.

Some of the questions to consider are:

- Do you want to have children?
- Is your pain intermittent, just around your periods?
- Does chronic pain prevent you from carrying out your daily activities?
- Are you nearing menopause, when adenomyosis related symptoms may go away?

Conclusion

In summary, it is so important that you understand your body. Tracking your cycle will help you to understand symptoms, flows, irregularities, and anything else that could be up with the body. If the body isn't working the way we want then it's trying to tell you something. The recommendation is always to seek medical advice if you are unsure or worried about anything.

Symptoms happen for a reason and there are treatments and interventions that can be made.

If you are unsure, please talk to your doctor for more guidance. If you are unhappy with the answer, please do not be afraid to ask for a second opinion.

For any nutritional guidance, doctors may not be able to provide the most up to date information, through no fault of their own, the education system needs improving in order to be able to provide the best possible advice for those who may be struggling.

Please work with a Nutritionist or a Dietitian for guidance.

Conclusion

Every woman is different and has the right to understand how their body works for them.

No one can pressure any woman to make a choice that they are not comfortable with. This could be anything from going on the pill, managing PCOS/Endometriosis, managing your perimenopause/Menopause.

It doesn't matter what stage you are at in your life the biggest thing to realise is:

"It's not your fault"

There is so much change that goes on for a woman and unfortunately not enough education or enough people talking about the female body and how it works. Over 51% of the world are female so it is time to know once and for all on how to manage your body for you.

The advice in this book does not replace any medical advice so if you have something underlying, never feel like you are annoying anyone, it's your body and you have the right to know what's going on in your body and mind.

The last thing I will say in this book is please spread the word in this book and share it with your friends and even your PT in the gym. This book is for every woman that is out there that wants to know what is going on with their body.

You got this!

References:

The references in this book are from a variety of sources and appear in order of appearance in the book itself.

Chapter 1 - The Cycle

Sung E, Han A, Hinrichs T, Vorgerd M, Manchado C, Platen P. Effects of follicular versus luteal phase-based strength training in young women. Springerplus. 2014 Dec 1;3(1):668.

Wikström-Frisén L, Boraxbekk CJ, Henriksson-Larsén K. Effects on power, strength and lean body mass of menstrual/oral contraceptive cycle based resistance training. Journal of Sports Medicine and Physical Fitness. 2015.

Reis E, Frick U, Schmidtbleicher D. Frequency variations of strength training sessions triggered by the phases of the menstrual cycle. International journal of sports medicine. 1995 Nov;16(08):545–50.

Herzberg SD, Motu'apuaka ML, Lambert W, Fu R, Brady J, Guise JM. The effect of menstrual cycle and contraceptives on ACL injuries and laxity: a systematic review and meta-analysis. Orthopaedic journal of sports medicine. 2017 Jul 19;5(7):2325967117718781.

Tacani PM, Ribeiro Dde O, Barros Guimarães BE, Machado AF, Tacani RE. Characterization of symptoms and edema distribution in premenstrual syndrome. Int J Womens Health. 2015 Mar

11;7:297-303. doi: 10.2147/IJWH.S74251. PMID: 25792857; PMCID: PMC4362892.

Chapter 2 - PMS & Cravings

Winer, S. A., Rapkin, A. J. (2006). Premenstrual disorders: prevalence, etiology and impact. Journal of Reproductive Medicine; 51(4 Suppl):339-347.

Dennerstein, L., Lehert, P., Heinemann, K. (2011). Global study of women's experiences of premenstrual symptoms and their effects on daily life. Menopause International; 17: 88–95.

WENDY S. BIGGS, MD, American Academy of Family Physicians, Leawood, Kansas ROBIN H. DEMUTH, MD, Michigan State University College of Human Medicine, East Lansing, Michigan
Am Fam Physician. 2011 Oct 15;84(8):918-924.

Wildpower - by ALEXANDRA POPE and SJANIE HUGO WURLITZER Discover the Magic of Your Menstrual Cycle and Awaken the Feminine Path to Power (Hay House, 2017)

Yonkers KA, O'Brien PMS, Eriksson E. Premenstrual syndrome. Lancet. 2008 Apr 5;371(9619):1200–10.

Bertone-Johnson ER, Hankinson SE, Bendich A, Johnson SR, Willett WC, Manson JE. Calcium and vitamin D intake and risk of incident premenstrual syndrome. Arch Intern Med. 2005 Jun 13;165(11):1246–52.

Chocano-Bedoya PO, Manson JE, Hankinson SE, Willett WC, Johnson SR, Chasan-Taber L, et al. Dietary B vitamin intake and incident premenstrual syndrome. The American Journal of Clinical Nutrition. 2011 May 1;93(5):1080–6.

Mohebbi Dehnavi Z, Jafarnejad F, Sadeghi Goghary S. The effect of 8 weeks aerobic exercise on severity of physical symptoms of premenstrual syndrome: a clinical trial study. BMC Womens Health. 2018 31;18(1):80.

Wu W-L, Lin T-Y, Chu I-H, Liang J-M. The Acute Effects of Yoga on Cognitive Measures for Women with Premenstrual Syndrome. The Journal of Alternative and Complementary Medicine. 2015 Jun;21(6):364–9.

Kjellgren A, Bood SÅ, Axelsson K, Norlander T, Saatcioglu F. Wellness through a comprehensive Yogic breathing program – A controlled pilot trial. BMC Complement Altern Med. 2007 Dec;7(1):43.

Bluth K, Gaylord S, Nguyen K, Bunevicius A, Girdler S. Mindfulness-based Stress Reduction as a Promising Intervention for Amelioration of Premenstrual Dysphoric Disorder Symptoms. Mindfulness (N Y). 2015 Dec;6(6):1292–302.

Lustyk MKB, Gerrish WG, Shaver S, Keys SL. Cognitive-behavioral therapy for premenstrual syndrome and premenstrual dysphoric disorder: a systematic review. Arch Womens Ment Health. 2009 Apr;12(2):85–96.

DiNicolantonio JJ, O'Keefe JH, Wilson W. Subclinical magnesium deficiency: a principal driver of cardiovascular disease and a public health crisis. Open Heart. 2018 Jan;5(1):e000668.

Fathizadeh N, Ebrahimi E, Valiani M, Tavakoli N, Yar MH. Evaluating the effect of magnesium and magnesium plus vitamin B6 supplement on the severity of premenstrual syndrome. Iran J Nurs Midwifery Res. 2010 Dec;15(Suppl 1):401–5.

Romans SE, Kreindler D, Asllani E, Einstein G, Laredo S, Levitt A, et al. Mood and the Menstrual Cycle. Psychother Psychosom. 2013;82(1):53–60.

Mortola JF. Issues in the diagnosis and research of premenstrual syndrome. Clin Obstet Gynecol. 1992 Sep;35(3):587–98.

Cerqueira RO, Frey BN, Leclerc E, Brietzke E. Vitex agnus castus for premenstrual syndrome and premenstrual dysphoric disorder: a systematic review. Arch Womens Ment Health. 2017 Dec;20(6):713-719. doi: 10.1007/s00737-017-0791-0. Epub 2017 Oct 23. PMID: 29063202.

Carmichael AR. Can Vitex Agnus Castus be Used for the Treatment of Mastalgia? What is the Current Evidence? Evid Based Complement Alternat Med. 2008 Sep;5(3):247-50. doi: 10.1093/ecam/nem074. PMID: 18830450; PMCID: PMC2529385.

Wuttke W, Jarry H, Christoffel V, Spengler B, Seidlová-Wuttke D. Chaste tree (Vitex agnus-castus)--pharmacology and clinical indications. Phytomedicine. 2003 May;10(4):348-57. doi: 10.1078/094471103322004866. PMID: 12809367.

Huddleston M, Jackson EA. Is an extract of the fruit of agnus castus (chaste tree or chasteberry) effective for prevention of symptoms of premenstrual syndrome (PMS)? J Fam Pract. 2001 Apr;50(4):298. PMID: 11300976.

Schellenberg R. Treatment for the premenstrual syndrome with agnus castus fruit extract: prospective, randomised, placebo controlled study. BMJ. 2001 Jan 20;322(7279):134-7. doi: 10.1136/bmj.322.7279.134. PMID: 11159568; PMCID: PMC26589.

Loch EG, Selle H, Boblitz N. Treatment of premenstrual syndrome with a phytopharmaceutical formulation containing Vitex agnus castus. J Womens Health Gend Based Med. 2000 Apr;9(3):315-20. doi: 10.1089/152460900318515. PMID: 10787228.

El-Lithy A, El-Mazny A, Sabbour A, El-Deeb A. Effect of aerobic exercise on premenstrual symptoms, haematological and hormonal parameters in young women. J Obstet Gynaecol. 2015 May;35(4):389-92. doi: 10.3109/01443615.2014.960823. Epub 2014 Oct 3. PMID: 25279689.

Fernández MDM, Saulyte J, Inskip HM, Takkouche B. BMJ Open. 2018 Apr 16;8(3):e019490

Eagon PK. Alcoholic liver injury: Influence of gender and hormones. World J Gastroenterol. 2010 Mar 21; 16(11): 1377–1384.

Becker U. The influence of ethanol and liver disease on sex hormones and hepatic oestrogen receptors in women. Dan Med Bull. 1993 Sep;40(4):447–59.

Becker U, Tønnesen H, Kaas-Claesson N, Gluud C.Menstrual disturbances and fertility in chronic alcoholic women. Drug Alcohol Depend. 1989 Aug;24(1):75–82.

Schliep KC, Zarek SM, Schisterman EF, Wactawski-Wende J, Trevisan M, Sjaarda LA, Perkins NJ, Mumford SL. Alcohol intake, reproductive hormones, and menstrual cycle function: a prospective cohort study. Am J Clin Nutr. 2015 Oct;102(4):933–42.

Lyngso J, Toft G, Hoyer BB, Guldbrandsen K, Olsen J, Ramlau-Hansen CH. Moderate alcohol intake and menstrual cycle characteristics. Hum Reprod. 2014;29(2):351–8.

Evans SM, Levin FR. Response to alcohol in women: role of the menstrual cycle and a family history of alcoholism. Drug Alcohol Depend. 2011;114(1):18–30.

Carroll HA, Lustyk KB, Larimer ME. The relationship between alcohol consumption and menstrual cycle: a review of the literature. Arch Womens Ment Health. 2015 Dec; 18(6): 773–781.

Tate DL, Charette L. Personality, alcohol

consumption, and menstrual distress in young women. Alcohol Clin Exp Res. 1991 Aug;15(4):647–52.

Gill J. The effects of moderate alcohol consumption on female hormone levels and reproductive function. Alcohol and Alcoholism. 2000 Sep 1;35(5):417–23.

Reichman ME, Judd JT, Longcope C, Schatzkin A, Clevidence BA, Nair PP, Campbell WS, Taylor PR. Effects of alcohol consumption on plasma and urinary hormone concentrations in premenopausal women. Natl Cancer Inst. 1993 May 5;85(9):722–7.

Dunn W, Shah VH. Pathogenesis of Alcoholic Liver Disease. Clin Liver Dis. 2016 Aug;20(3):445–456.

Menon KV, Gores GJ, Shah VH. Pathogenesis, diagnosis, and treatment of alcoholic liver disease. Mayo Clin Proc. 2001 Oct;76(10):1021–9.

Bertha J. Vandegrift, Chang You, Rosalba Satta, Mark S. Brodie, Amy W. Lasek. Estradiol increases the sensitivity of ventral tegmental area dopamine neurons to dopamine and ethanol. PLOS ONE, 2017;12(11): e0187698.
Torgerson DJ, Thomas RE, Campbell MK, Reid DM. Alcohol consumption and age of maternal menopause are associated with menopause onset. Maturitas. 1997 Jan;26(1):21–5.

Taneri PE, Kiefte-de Jong JC, Bramer WM, Daan NM, Franco OH, Muka T. Association of alcohol consumption with the onset of natural menopause: a systematic review and meta-analysis.Hum Reprod

Update. 2016 Jun;22(4):516–28.

Fan D, Liu L, Xia Q, Wang W, Wu S, Tian G, Liu Y, Ni J, Wu S, Guo X, Liu Z. Female alcohol consumption and fecundability: a systematic review and dose-response meta-analysis. Sci Rep. 2017 Oct 23;7(1):13815.

Homan GF, Davies M, Norman R. The impact of lifestyle factors on reproductive performance in the general population and those undergoing infertility treatment: a review. Hum Reprod Update. 2007 May-Jun;13(3):209–23.

The American College of Obstetricians and Gynecologists. FAQ: Premenstrual syndrome. 2015. Retrieved from http://www.acog.org/~/media/For%20Patients/faq057.pdf?

Rossignol, A.M. (1985). Caffeine-containing beverages and premenstrual syndrome in young women. Am J Public Health, 75,1335–7.

Rossignol AM, Zhang J, Chen Y, Xiang Z. (1989). Tea and premenstrual syndrome in the People's Republic of China. Am J Public Health, 79, 67–9.

Rossignol A.M. & Bonnlander, H. (1990). Caffeine-containing beverages, total fluid consumption, and premenstrual syndrome. Am J Public Health, 80,1106–10.

Rossignol, A., Bonnlander, H., Song, L., & Phillis, J. (1991). Do women with premenstrual symptoms self-medicate with caffeine? Epidemiology, 2(6), 403–408. Retrieved from http://www.jstor.org/stable/20065717

Chayachinda, C., Rattanachaiyanont, M., Phattharayuttawat, S., & Kooptiwoot, S. (2008). Premenstrual syndrome in Thai nurses. Journal of Psychosomatic Obstetrics & Gynecology, 29(3), 203–209. doi:10.1080/01674820801970306

Caan, B., Duncan, D., Hiatt, R., Lewis, J., Chapman, J., & Armstrong, M.A. (1993). Association between alcoholic and caffeinated beverages and premenstrual syndrome. J Reprod Med, 38, 630–6.

Gold E.B., Bair Y., Block G., Greendale G.A., Harlow S.D., Johnson S., Kravitz H.M., Rasor M.O., Siddiqui A., Sternfeld B., et al. (2007). Diet and lifestyle factors associated with premenstrual symptoms in a racially diverse community sample: Study of Women's Health Across the Nation (SWAN). Journal of Women's Health (Larchmt), 6, 641–56.

Vo, H., Smith, B., & Rubinow, D. (2010). Effects of caffeine consumption on premenstrual syndrome: a prospective study. Internet Journal of Endocrinology, 6,1–6.

Purdue-Smithe A.C., Manson J.E., Hankinson S.E., & Bertone-Johnson E.R. (2016). A prospective study of caffeine and coffee intake and premenstrual syndrome. American Journal of Clinical Epidemiology. doi: 10.3945/ajcn.115.127027 14.

Biggs, W. S., & Demuth, R. H. (2011). Premenstrual syndrome and premenstrual dysphoric disorder. American Family Physician, 84(8).

Noreika, D., Griškova-Bulanova, I., Alaburda, A., Baranauskas, M., & Grikšienė, R. (2014). Progesterone and mental rotation task: is there any effect? BioMed Research International. http://www.ncbi.nlm.nih.gov/pubmed/24818150

N. Rahbar et al. / International Journal of Gynecology and Obstetrics 117 (2012) 45–47 Curcumin attenuates severity of premenstrual syndrome symptoms: A randomized, double-blind, placebo-controlled trial. Complementary Therapies in Medicine Volume 23, Issue 3, June 2015, Pages 318-324

Fathizadeh N, Ebrahimi E, Valiani M, Tavakoli N, Yar MH. Evaluating the effect of magnesium and magnesium plus vitamin B6 supplement on the severity of premenstrual syndrome. Iran J Nurs Midwifery Res. 2010 Dec;15(Suppl 1):401-5. PMID: 22069417; PMCID: PMC3208934.

Saeedian Kia A, Amani R, Cheraghian B. The Association between the Risk of Premenstrual Syndrome and Vitamin D, Calcium, and Magnesium Status among University Students: A Case Control Study. Health Promot Perspect. 2015 Oct 25;5(3):225-30. doi: 10.15171/hpp.2015.027. Erratum in: Health Promot Perspect. 2016;6(1):54. PMID: 26634201; PMCID: PMC4667262.

Masoumi SZ, Asl HR, Poorolajal J, Panah MH,

Oliaei SR. Evaluation of mint efficacy regarding dysmenorrhea in comparison with mefenamic acid: A double blinded randomized crossover study. Iranian J Nursing Midwifery Res 2016;21:363-7

Valiani M, Ghasemi N, Bahadoran P, Heshmat R. The effects of massage therapy on dysmenorrhea caused by endometriosis. Iran J Nurs Midwifery Res. 2010 Fall;15(4):167-71. PMID: 21589790; PMCID: PMC3093183.

Hormes JM, Niemiec MA (2017) Does culture create craving? Evidence from the case of menstrual chocolate craving. PLoS ONE 12(7): e0181445. https://doi.org/10.1371/journal.pone.0181445

Cleveland Clinic

Romans S, Clarkson R, Einstein G, Petrovic M, Stewart D. Mood and the menstrual cycle: a review of prospective data studies. Gend Med. 2012;9(5):361–84.

American College of Obstetricians and Gynecologists. Premenstrual Syndrome (PMS) [Internet]. Premenstrual Syndrome (PMS). 2015. Available from: https://www.acog.org/patient-resources/faqs/gynecologic-problems/premenstrual-syndrome

Tharpe N, Farley CL, Jordan RG. Clinical practice guidelines for midwifery and women's health. 4th ed. Burlington, Mass: Jones & Bartlett Learning; 2013. 622 p.415

Johnson SR. The epidemiology and social impact of premenstrual symptoms. Clinical Obstetrics and Gynecology. 1987 Jun;30(2):367–76.

Cheng SH, Sun ZJ, Lee IH, Shih CC, Chen KC, Lin SH, et al. Perception of premenstrual syndrome and attitude of evaluations of work performance among incoming university female students. Biomed J. 2015;38(2):167–72.

Walker A. Theory and methodology in premenstrual syndrome research. Soc Sci Med. 1995;41(6):793–800.

Roos J, Johnson S, Weddell S, Godehardt E, Schiffner J, Freundl G, et al. Monitoring the menstrual cycle: Comparison of urinary and serum reproductive hormones referenced to true ovulation. Eur J Contracept Reprod Health Care. 2015:1–13.

Rapkin AJ, Mikacich JA. Premenstrual syndrome and premenstrual dysphoric disorder in adolescents. Curr Opin Obstet Gynecol. 2008;20(5):455–63.

Frackiewicz EJ, Shiovitz TM. Evaluation and management of premenstrual syndrome and premenstrual dysphoric disorder. J Am Pharm Assoc (Wash). 2001;41(3):437–47.

Jarvis CI, Lynch AM, Morin AK. Management strategies for premenstrual syndrome/premenstrual dysphoric disorder. Ann Pharmacother. 2008;42(7):967–78.

Lauersen NH. Recognition and treatment of

premenstrual syndrome. Nurse Pract. 1985;10(3):11–2, 5, 8–20.

Romans SE, Kreindler D, Asllani E, Einstein G, Laredo S, Levitt A, et al. Mood and the menstrual cycle. Psychother Psychosom. 2013;82(1):53–60.

Kikuchi H, Nakatani Y, Seki Y, Yu X, Sekiyama T, Sato-Suzuki I, et al. Decreased blood serotonin in the premenstrual phase enhances negative mood in healthy women. J Psychosom Obstet Gynaecol. 2010;31(2):83–9.

Chapter 3 - The Pill

Sulak PJ, Cressman BE, Waldrop E, Holleman S, Kuehl TJ. Extending the duration of active oral contraceptive pills to manage hormone withdrawal symptoms. Obstetrics & Gynecology. 1997 Feb 1;89(2):179-83.

Johnson JV, Grubb GS, Constantine GD. Endometrial histology following 1 year of a continuous daily regimen of levonorgestrel 90 µg/ethinyl estradiol 20 µg. Contraception. 2007 Jan 31;75(1):23-6.

Wright KP, Johnson JV. Evaluation of extended and continuous use oral contraceptives. 2008

Lyle McDonalds work in particular, the Women's Book Vol 1: A guide to Nutrition, Fat loss and Muscle Gain.

NHS

Li CI, Beaber EF, Tang MT, Porter PL, Daling JR, Malone KE. Effect of depo-medroxyprogesterone acetate on breast cancer risk among women 20 to 44 years of age. Cancer Res. 2012 Apr 15;72(8):2028-35. doi: 10.1158/0008-5472.CAN-11-4064. Epub 2012 Feb 27. PMID: 22369929; PMCID: PMC3328650.

Kailasam C, Cahill D. Review of the safety, efficacy and patient acceptability of the levonorgestrel-releasing intrauterine system. Patient Prefer Adherence. 2008 Feb 2;2:293-302. doi: 10.2147/ppa.s3464. PMID: 19920976; PMCID: PMC2770406.

Mayo Clinic

Skovlund CW, Mørch LS, Kessing LV, Lidegaard Ø. Association of Hormonal Contraception With Depression. JAMA Psychiatry. 2016 Nov 1;73(11):1154-1162. doi: 10.1001/jamapsychiatry.2016.2387. Erratum in: JAMA Psychiatry. 2017 Jul 1;74(7):764. PMID: 27680324.

Aleknaviciute J, Tulen JHM, De Rijke YB, Bouwkamp CG, van der Kroeg M, Timmermans M, Wester VL, Bergink V, Hoogendijk WJG, Tiemeier H, van Rossum EFC, Kooiman CG, Kushner SA. The levonorgestrel-releasing intrauterine device potentiates stress reactivity. Psychoneuroendocrinology. 2017 Jun;80:39-45. doi: 10.1016/j.psyneuen.2017.02.025. Epub 2017 Feb 28. PMID: 28315609.

Samira Khayat, Hamed Fanaei, Masoomeh Kheirkhah, Zahra Behboodi Moghadam, Amir Kasaeian, Mani Javadimehr, Curcumin attenuates severity of premenstrual syndrome symptoms: A randomized, double-blind, placebo-controlled trial, Complementary Therapies in Medicine, Volume 23, Issue 3, 2015, Pages 318-324, ISSN 0965-2299, https://doi.org/10.1016/j.ctim.2015.04.001.

Böttcher, B., Radenbach, K., Wildt, L. et al. Hormonal contraception and depression: a survey of the present state of knowledge. Arch Gynecol Obstet 286, 231–236 (2012). https://doi.org/10.1007/s00404-012-2298-2

Mental Health America - https://www.mhanational.org/depression-women

Higgins JA, Smith NK. The sexual acceptability of contraception: reviewing the literature and building a new concept. J Sex Res. 2016 May 3;53(4-5):417-56.

Pastor Z, Holla K, Chmel R. The influence of combined oral contraceptives on female sexual desire: a systematic review. Eur J Contracept Reprod Health Care. 2013;18(1):27–43.

Latif EZ, Diamond MP. Arriving at the diagnosis of female sexual dysfunction. Fertil Steril. 2013 Oct 31;100(4):898–904.

American College of Obstetricians and Gynecologists. Female sexual dysfunction. ACOG

Practice Bulletin №119. Obstet Gynecol. 2011;117(4):996–1007.

Safarinejad MR. Female sexual dysfunction in a population-based study in Iran: prevalence and associated risk factors. Int J Impot Res. 2006 Jul 1;18(4):382–95.

Emhardt E, Siegel J, Hoffman L. Anatomic variation and orgasm: could variations in anatomy explain differences in orgasmic success?. Clin Anat. 2016 Jul 1;29(5):665–72.

Rivera R, Yacobson I, Grimes D. The mechanism of action of hormonal contraceptives and intrauterine contraceptive devices. Am J Obstet Gynecol. 1999;181(5):1263–9.

Zethraeus N, Dreber A, Ranehill E, Blomberg L, Labrie F, von Schoultz B, et al. Combined oral contraceptives and sexual function in women—a double-blind, randomized, placebo-controlled trial. J Clin Endocrinol Metab. 2016 Aug 15;101(11):4046-53.

Parish SJ, Hahn SR. Hypoactive sexual desire disorder: a review of epidemiology, biopsychology, diagnosis, and treatment. Sex Med Rev. 2016 Apr 1;4(2):103-20.

Elsenbruch S, Hahn S, Kowalsky D, Offner AH, Schedlowski M, Mann K, et al. Quality of life, psychosocial well-being and sexual satisfaction in women with polycystic ovary syndrome. J Clin Endocrinol Metab 2003;88:5801–7.

Shifren JL, Braunstein GD, Simon JA, Casson PR, Buster JE, Redmond GP, et al. Transdermal testosterone treatment in women with impaired sexual function after oophorectomy. New Engl J Med 2000;343:682-8.

Roumen FJ. Review of the combined contraceptive vaginal ring, NuvaRing®. Ther Clin Risk Manag. 2008 Apr;4(2):441.

Guida M, Cibarelli F, Troisi J, Gallo A, Palumbo AR, Sardo AD. Sexual life impact evaluation of different hormonal contraceptives on the basis of their methods of administration. Arch Gynecol Obstet. 2014 Dec 1;290(6):1239-47.

American College of Obstetricians and Gynecologists. ACOG Practice Bulletin №110: noncontraceptive uses of hormonal contraceptives. Obstet Gynecol. 2010;115(1):206–18.

American College of Obstetricians and Gynecologists. ACOG FAQ186: Progestin-Only Hormonal Birth Control: Pill and Injection. 2018. Available from: https://www.acog.org/Patients/FAQs/Progestin-Only-Hormonal-Birth-Control-Pill-and-Injection

Elaut E, Buysse A, De Sutter P, De Cuypere G, Gerris J, Deschepper E, et al. Relation of androgen receptor sensitivity and mood to sexual desire in hormonal contraception users. Contraception. 2012 May 1;85(5):470-9.

Graham CA, Ramos R, Bancroft J, Maglaya C,

Farley TM. The effects of steroidal contraceptives on the well-being and sexuality of women: a double-blind, placebo-controlled, two-centre study of combined and progestogen-only methods. Contraception. 1995 Dec 1;52(6):363-9.

Boozalis MA, Tutlam NT, Robbins CC, Peipert JF. Sexual desire and hormonal contraception. Obstet Gynecol. 2016 Mar;127(3):563-72.

Wanyonyi SZ, Stones WR, Sequeira E. Health-related quality of life changes among users of depot medroxyprogesterone acetate for contraception. Contraception. 2011 Nov 1;84(5):e17-22.

Ott MA, Shew ML, Ofner S, Tu W, Fortenberry JD. The influence of hormonal contraception on mood and sexual interest among adolescents. Arch Sex Behav. 2008 Aug 1;37(4):605-13.

Schaffir JA, Isley MM, Woodward M. Oral contraceptives vs injectable progestin in their effect on sexual behavior. Am J Obstet Gynecol. 2010 Dec 1;203(6):545-e1.

Hatcher RA, Nelson AL, Trussell J, et al. Contraceptive Technology (21st edition). New York :Ayer Company Publishers. 2018.

Aisien AO, Enosolease ME. Safety, efficacy and acceptability of implanon a single rod implantable contraceptive (etonogestrel) in University of Benin Teaching Hospital. Niger J Clin Pract. 2010 Sep;13(3):331-5.

Gezginc K, Balci O, Karatayli R, Colakoglu MC. Contraceptive efficacy and side effects of Implanon®. Eur J Contracept Reprod Health Care. 2007 Jan 1;12(4):362-5.

Duvan Cİ, Gözdemir E, Kaygusuz İ, Kamalak Z, Turhan NÖ. Etonogestrel contraceptive implant (Implanon): analysis of patient compliance and adverse effects in the breastfeeding period. J Turk Ger Gynecol Assoc. 2010 Sep 1;11(3):141-4.

Bitzer J, Tschudin S, Alder J, Swiss Implanon Study Group. Acceptability and side-effects of Implanon in Switzerland: a retrospective study by the Implanon Swiss Study Group. The Eur J Contracept Reprod Health Care. 2004 Jan 1;9(4):278-84.

Brache V, Faundes A, Alvarez F, Cochon L. Nonmenstrual adverse events during use of implantable contraceptives for women: data from clinical trials. Contraception. 2002 Jan 1;65(1):63-74.

Di Carlo C, Sansone A, De Rosa N, Gargano V, Tommaselli GA, Nappi C, et al. Impact of an implantable steroid contraceptive (etonogestrel-releasing implant) on quality of life and sexual function: a preliminary study. Gynecol Endocrinol. 2014 Jan 1;30(1):53-6.

Trussell J. Contraceptive failure in the United States. Contraception. 2011 May 1;83(5):397-404.

Oddens BJ. Women's satisfaction with birth control: a population survey of physical and psychological effects of oral contraceptives, intrauterine devices, condoms, natural family planning, and sterilization among 1466 women. Contraception. 1999 May 1;59(5):277-86.

Bastianelli C, Farris M, Benagiano G. Use of the levonorgestrel-releasing intrauterine system, quality of life and sexuality. Experience in an Italian family planning center. Contraception. 2011 Oct 1;84(4):402-8.

Skrzypulec V, Drosdzol A. Evaluation of quality of life and sexual functioning of women using levonorgestrel-releasing intrauterine contraceptive system–Mirena. Coll Antropol. 2008 Dec 1;32(4):1059-68.

Enzlin P, Weyers S, Janssens D, Poppe W, Eelen C, Pazmany E, et al. Sexual functioning in women using levonorgestrel-releasing intrauterine systems as compared to copper intrauterine devices. J Sex Med. 2012 Apr 1;9(4):1065-73.

www.helloclue.com

Scholes D, Hubbard RA, Ichikawa LE, LaCroix AZ, Spangler L, Beasley JM, Reed S, Ott SM. Oral contraceptive use and bone density change in adolescent and young adult women: a prospective study of age, hormone dose, and discontinuation. J Clin Endocrinol Metab. 2011 Sep;96(9):E1380-7. doi: 10.1210/jc.2010-3027. Epub 2011 Jul 13. PMID: 21752879; PMCID: PMC3167673.

Scholes D, Ichikawa L, LaCroix AZ, Spangler L,

Beasley JM, Reed S, Ott SM. Oral contraceptive use and bone density in adolescent and young adult women. Contraception. 2010 Jan;81(1):35-40. doi: 10.1016/j.contraception.2009.07.001. PMID: 20004271; PMCID: PMC2822656.

Sulak PJ, Cressman BE, Waldrop E, Holleman S, Kuehl TJ. Extending the duration of active oral contraceptive pills to manage hormone withdrawal symptoms. Obstetrics & Gynecology. 1997 Feb 1;89(2):179-83.

Johnson JV, Grubb GS, Constantine GD. Endometrial histology following 1 year of a continuous daily regimen of levonorgestrel 90 µg/ethinyl estradiol 20 µg. Contraception. 2007 Jan 31;75(1):23-6.

Wright KP, Johnson JV. Evaluation of extended and continuous use oral contraceptives. 2008

Lyle McDonalds work in particular, the Women's Book Vol 1: A guide to Nutrition, Fat loss and Muscle Gain.

Chapter 4 - Hypothalamic Amenorrhea (HA)

Sarah Liz King - Holistic health radio Podcast

No Period Now What - Dr. Nicola Rinaldi

Chapter 5 - PCOS

Jamilian M, et al. (2016). Effects of zinc supplementation on endocrine outcomes in women with polycystic ovary syndrome: A randomized, double-blind, placebo-controlled trial. DOI: 10.1007/s12011-015-0480-7

Moran LJ, et al. (2011). Lifestyle changes in women with polycystic ovary syndrome. DOI: 10.1002/14651858.CD007506.pub2

Ablon G. (2015). A 3-month, randomized, double-blind, placebo-controlled study evaluating the ability of an extra-strength marine protein supplement to promote hair growth and decrease shedding in women with self-perceived thinning hair. DOI: 10.1155/2015/841570

Herskovitz I, et al. (2013). Female pattern hair loss. DOI: 10.5812/ijem.9860 Consensus on women's health aspects of polycystic ovary syndrome (PCOS). (2012). DOI: 10.1093/humrep/der396

Indian J Dermatol. 2010 HIRSUTISM: EVALUATION AND TREATMENT
doi: 10.4103/0019-5154.60342

Lara briden, Period repair Manual

Pasquapina Ciarmela and Fabio Parazzin (2021): Nutrition Strategy and Life Style in Polycystic Ovary Syndrome—Narrative Review
Nutrients 2021,, 2452; https://doi.org/10.3390/nu13072452

J Turk Ger Gynecol Assoc. (2018); The effect of nutrient supplementation in the management of polycystic ovary syndrome-associated metabolic dysfunctions: A critical review doi: 10.4274/jtgga.2018.0077

Wei Wei , Hongmin Zhao, Aili Wang, Ming Sui, Kun Liang, Haiyun Deng, Yukun Ma, Yajuan Zhang, Hongxiu Zhang, Yuanyuan Guan: A clinical study on the short-term effect of berberine in comparison to metformin on the metabolic characteristics of women with polycystic ovary syndrome, DOI: 10.1530/EJE-11-0616, PMID: 22019891

JBRA Assist Reprod. 2019 Effects of L-carnitine on Polycystic Ovary Syndrome doi: 10.5935/1518-0557.20190033 PMID: 31294953

Young Sun Kim and Nayoung Kim, 2020: Sex-Gender Differences in Irritable Bowel Syndrome: doi: 10.5056/jnm18082   PMID: 30347934

Senthurselvi Ramamoorthy and Bhuvaneswari K (2019); A Cross Sectional Study on the Status of Inflammatory Markers in Polycystic Ovary Syndrome (Pcos) in Indian Population DOI : https://dx.doi.org/10.13005/bpj/1829

Healthline: www.healthline.com

Nikokavoura EA, Johnston KL, Broom J, Wrieden WL, Rolland C. Weight loss for women with and without polycystic ovary syndrome following a very low-calorie diet in a community-based setting with trained facilitators for 12 weeks. Diabetes Metab

Syndr Obes. 2015 Oct 14;8:495-503. doi: 10.2147/DMSO.S85134. PMID: 26508882; PMCID: PMC4610794.

Examine.com

Shukla KK, Mahdi AA, Ahmad MK, Shankhwar SN, Rajender S, Jaiswar SP. Mucuna pruriens improves male fertility by its action on the hypothalamus-pituitary-gonadal axis. Fertil Steril. 2009 Dec;92(6):1934-40. doi: 10.1016/j.fertnstert.2008.09.045. Epub 2008 Oct 29. PMID: 18973898.

Barletta C, Sellini M, Bartoli A, Bigi C, Buzzetti R, Giovannini C. Influenza della somministrazione di piridossina sul ritmo circadiano dell'acth, del cortisolo, della prolattina e del somatotropo plasmatici nei soggetti normali [Influence of administration of pyridoxine on circadian rhythm of plasma ACTH, cortisol prolactin and somatotropin in normal subjects]. Boll Soc Ital Biol Sper. 1984 Feb 28;60(2):273-8. Italian. PMID: 6324828.

Lepore E, Lauretta R, Bianchini M, Mormando M, Di Lorenzo C, Unfer V. Inositols Depletion and Resistance: Principal Mechanisms and Therapeutic Strategies. International Journal of Molecular Sciences. 2021;22(13):6796.

Unfer V, Porcaro G. Updates on the myo-inositol plus D-chiro-inositol combined therapy in polycystic ovary syndrome. Expert Review of Clinical Pharmacology. 2014;7(5):623-631.

Iuorno M, Jakubowicz D, Baillargeon J, Dillon P, Gunn R, Allan G et al. Effects of D-Chiro-Inositol in Lean Women with the Polycystic Ovary Syndrome. Endocrine Practice. 2002;8(6):417-423.

Wei W, Zhao H, Wang A, Sui M, Liang K, Deng H et al. A clinical study on the short-term effect of berberine in comparison to metformin on the metabolic characteristics of women with polycystic ovary syndrome. European Journal of Endocrinology. 2012;166(1):99-105.

NHS

Kalem MN, Kalem Z, Sarı T, Ateş C, Gürgan T. Effect of body mass index and age on in vitro fertilization in polycystic ovary syndrome. J Turk Ger Gynecol Assoc. 2016 Jan 12;17(2):83-90. doi: 10.5152/jtgga.2016.15235. PMID: 27403074; PMCID: PMC4922730.

Kalem MN, Kalem Z, Sarı T, Ateş C, Gürgan T. Effect of body mass index and age on in vitro fertilization in polycystic ovary syndrome. J Turk Ger Gynecol Assoc. 2016 Jan 12;17(2):83-90. doi: 10.5152/jtgga.2016.15235. PMID: 27403074; PMCID: PMC4922730.

Chapter 6 - Endometriosis

Bailey LB, Caudill MA. Folate. In: Erdman JW, Macdonald IA, Zeisel SH, eds. Present Knowledge in Nutrition. 10th ed. Washington, DC: Wiley-Blackwell; 2012:321-42.

Institute of Medicine. Food and Nutrition Board. Dietary Reference Intakes: Thiamin, Riboflavin, Niacin, Vitamin B6, Folate, Vitamin B12, Pantothenic Acid, Biotin, and Choline. Washington, DC: National Academy Press; 1998.

Stover PJ. Folic acid. In: Ross AC, Caballero B, Cousins RJ, Tucker KL, Ziegler TR, eds. Modern Nutrition in Health and Disease. 11th ed. Baltimore, MD: Lippincott Williams & Wilkins; 2012:358-68.

Carmel R. Folic acid. In: Shils M, Shike M, Ross A, Caballero B, Cousins RJ, eds. Modern Nutrition in Health and Disease. 11th ed. Baltimore, MD: Lippincott Williams & Wilkins; 2005:470-81.

Paniz C, Bertinato JF, Lucena MR, et al. A daily dose of 5 mg folic acid for 90 days is associated with increased serum unmetabolized folic acid and reduced natural killer cell cytotoxicity in healthy Brazilian adults. J Nutr 2017;147:1677-85.

Crider KS, Bailey LB, Berry RJ. Folic acid food fortification-its history, effect, concerns, and future directions. Nutrients 2011;3:370-84.

Yetley EA, Pfeiffer CM, Phinney KW, et al. Biomarkers of folate status in NHANES: a roundtable summary. Am J Clin Nutr 2011;94:303S-12S.

Lakoff A, Fazili Z, Aufreiter S, et al. Folate is absorbed across the human colon: evidence by using enteric-coated caplets containing 13C-labeled [6S]-5-formyltetrahydrofolate. Am J Clin Nutr 2014;100:1278-86.

Bailey LB, Stover PJ, McNulty H, et al. Biomarkers of nutrition for development-folate review. J Nutr 2015;145:1636S-80S.

Green R. Indicators for assessing folate and vitamin B-12 status and for monitoring the efficacy of intervention strategies. Am J Clin Nutr 2011;94:666S-72S.

U.S. Food and Drug Administration. Food Labeling: Revision of the Nutrition and Supplement Facts Labels. external link disclaimer2016.

U.S. Food and Drug Administration. Food Standards: Amendment of Standards of Identity For Enriched Grain Products to Require Addition of Folic Acid.external link disclaimer Federal Register 1996;61:8781-97.

Choumenkovitch SF, Selhub J, Wilson PW, et al. Folic acid intake from fortification in United States exceeds predictions. J Nutr 2002;132:2792-8.

U.S. Food and Drug Administration. FDA approves folic acid fortification of corn masa flour.external link disclaimer 2016.

Government of Canada. Regulations amending the food and drug regulations (1066). Canada Gazette 1998;132.

Centers for Disease Control and Prevention. CDC grand rounds: Additional opportunities to prevent neural tube defects with folic acid fortification.

MMWR Morb Mortal Wkly Rep 2010;59:980-4.

Yeung LF, Cogswell ME, Carriquiry AL, et al. Contributions of enriched cereal-grain products, ready-to-eat cereals, and supplements to folic acid and vitamin B-12 usual intake and folate and vitamin B-12 status in US children: National Health and Nutrition Examination Survey (NHANES), 2003-2006. Am J Clin Nutr 2011;93:172-85.

National Institutes of Health. Dietary Supplement Label Database. 2018.
Scaglione F, Panzavolta G. Folate, folic acid and 5-methyltetrahydrofolate are not the same thing. Xenobiotica 2014;44:480-8.

Greenberg JA, Bell SJ, Guan Y, et al. Folic acid supplementation and pregnancy: more than just neural tube defect prevention. Rev Obstet Gynecol 2011;4:52-9.

Henderson AM, Aleliunas RE, Loh SP, et al. l-5-Methyltetrahydrofolate supplementation increases blood folate concentrations to a greater extent than folic acid supplementation in Malaysian women. J Nutr 2018;148:885-90.

Green TJ, Liu Y, Dadgar S, et al. Wheat rolls fortified with microencapsulated L-5-methyltetrahydrofolic acid or equimolar folic acid increase blood folate concentrations to a similar extent in healthy men and women. J Nutr 2013;143:867-71.

Venn BJ, Green TJ, Moser R, et al. Comparison of

the effect of low-dose supplementation with L-5-methyltetrahydrofolate or folic acid on plasma homocysteine: a randomized placebo-controlled study. Am J Clin Nutr 2003;77:658-62.

Venn BJ, Green TJ, Moser R, et al. Increases in blood folate indices are similar in women of childbearing age supplemented with [6S]-5-methyltetrahydrofolate and folic acid. J Nutr 2002;132:3353-5.

Lamers Y, Prinz-Langenohl R, Bramswig S, et al. Red blood cell folate concentrations increase more after supplementation with [6S]-5-methyltetrahydrofolate than with folic acid in women of childbearing age. Am J Clin Nutr 2006;84:156-61.

Pietrzik K, Bailey L, Shane B. Folic acid and L-5-methyltetrahydrofolate: comparison of clinical pharmacokinetics and pharmacodynamics. Clin Pharmacokinet 2010;49:535-48.

U.S. Department of Agriculture, Agricultural Research Service. What We Eat in America, 2013-2014.external link disclaimer 2017.

Bailey RL, Dodd KW, Gahche JJ, et al. Total folate and folic acid intake from foods and dietary supplements in the United States: 2003-2006. Am J Clin Nutr 2010;91:231-7.

Bailey RL, McDowell MA, Dodd KW, et al. Total folate and folic acid intakes from foods and dietary supplements of US children aged 1-13 y. Am J Clin Nutr 2010;92:353-8.

Yang Q, Cogswell ME, Hamner HC, et al. Folic acid source, usual intake, and folate and vitamin B-12 status in US adults: National Health and Nutrition Examination Survey (NHANES) 2003-2006. Am J Clin Nutr 2010;91:64-72.

Ho RC, Cheung MW, Fu E, et al. Is high homocysteine level a risk factor for cognitive decline in elderly? A systematic review, meta-analysis, and meta-regression. Am J Geriatr Psychiatry 2011;19:607-17.

Scholl TO, Johnson WG. Folic acid: influence on the outcome of pregnancy. Am J Clin Nutr 2000;71:1295S-303S.

Gloria L, Cravo M, Camilo ME, et al. Nutritional deficiencies in chronic alcoholics: relation to dietary intake and alcohol consumption. Am J Gastroenterol 1997;92:485-9.

Gibson A, Woodside JV, Young IS, et al. Alcohol increases homocysteine and reduces B vitamin concentration in healthy male volunteers–a randomized, crossover intervention study. QJM 2008;101:881-7.

Centers for Disease Control and Prevention. Folic acid 2012.external link disclaimer
U. S. Preventive Services Task Force, Bibbins-Domingo K, Grossman DC, et al. Folic acid supplementation for the prevention of neural tube defects: US Preventive Services Task Force recommendation statement. JAMA 2017;317:183-9.

American College of Obstetricians and Gynecologists. Frequently Asked Questions, FAQ001, Pregnancy, Nutrition During Pregnancy.external link disclaimer 2018.
Rossi RE, Whyand T, Murray CD, et al. The role of dietary supplements in inflammatory bowel disease: a systematic review. Eur J Gastroenterol Hepatol 2016;28:1357-64.

Molloy AM, Pangilinan F, Brody LC. Genetic risk factors for folate-responsive neural tube defects. Annu Rev Nutr 2017;37:269-91.

National Institute of Mental Health. Autism spectrum disorder. 2018.
Berry RJ, Crider KS, Yeargin-Allsopp M. Periconceptional folic acid and risk of autism spectrum disorders. JAMA 2013;309:611-3.

Bjork M, Riedel B, Spigset O, et al. Association of folic acid supplementation during pregnancy with the risk of autistic traits in children exposed to antiepileptic drugs in utero. JAMA Neurol 2018;75:160-8.

Schmidt RJ, Kogan V, Shelton JF, et al. Combined prenatal pesticide exposure and folic acid intake in relation to autism spectrum disorder. Environ Health Perspect 2017;125:097007.

Goodrich AJ, Volk HE, Tancredi DJ, et al. Joint effects of prenatal air pollutant exposure and maternal folic acid supplementation on risk of autism spectrum disorder. Autism Res 2018;11:69-80.

Roffman JL. Neuroprotective effects of prenatal folic acid supplementation: why timing matters. JAMA Psychiatry 2018;75:747-8.

Caffrey A, Irwin RE, McNulty H, et al. Gene-specific DNA methylation in newborns in response to folic acid supplementation during the second and third trimesters of pregnancy: epigenetic analysis from a randomized controlled trial. Am J Clin Nutr 2018;107:566-75.

DeVilbiss EA, Gardner RM, Newschaffer CJ, et al. Maternal folate status as a risk factor for autism spectrum disorders: a review of existing evidence. Br J Nutr 2015;114:663-72.

Suren P, Roth C, Bresnahan M, et al. Association between maternal use of folic acid supplements and risk of autism spectrum disorders in children. JAMA 2013;309:570-7.

Schmidt RJ, Tancredi DJ, Ozonoff S, et al. Maternal periconceptional folic acid intake and risk of autism spectrum disorders and developmental delay in the CHARGE (CHildhood Autism Risks from Genetics and Environment) case-control study. Am J Clin Nutr 2012;96:80-9.

Levine SZ, Kodesh A, Viktorin A, et al. Association of maternal use of folic acid and multivitamin supplements in the periods before and during pregnancy with the risk of autism spectrum disorder in offspring. JAMA Psychiatry 2018;75:176-84.

Virk J, Liew Z, Olsen J, et al. Preconceptional and

prenatal supplementary folic acid and multivitamin intake and autism spectrum disorders. Autism 2016;20:710-8.

He H, Shui B. Folate intake and risk of bladder cancer: a meta-analysis of epidemiological studies. Int J Food Sci Nutr 2014;65:286-92.

Kim YI. Will mandatory folic acid fortification prevent or promote cancer? Am J Clin Nutr 2004;80:1123-8.

Kim YI. Folate and carcinogenesis: evidence, mechanisms, and implications. J Nutr Biochem 1999;10:66-88.

Kim YI. Folate and cancer: a tale of Dr. Jekyll and Mr. Hyde? Am J Clin Nutr 2018;107:139-42.

Andreeva VA, Touvier M, Kesse-Guyot E, et al. B vitamin and/or omega-3 fatty acid supplementation and cancer: ancillary findings from the supplementation with folate, vitamins B6 and B12, and/or omega-3 fatty acids (SU.FOL.OM3) randomized trial. Arch Intern Med 2012;172:540-7.

Ebbing M, Bonaa KH, Nygard O, et al. Cancer incidence and mortality after treatment with folic acid and vitamin B12. JAMA 2009;302:2119-26.

Mason JB. Unraveling the complex relationship between folate and cancer risk. Biofactors 2011;37:253-60.

Giovannucci E, Stampfer MJ, Colditz GA, et al. Folate, methionine, and alcohol intake and risk of colorectal adenoma. J Natl Cancer Inst 1993;85:875-84.

Gibson TM, Weinstein SJ, Pfeiffer RM, et al. Pre- and postfortification intake of folate and risk of colorectal cancer in a large prospective cohort study in the United States. Am J Clin Nutr 2011;94:1053-62.

Sanjoaquin MA, Allen N, Couto E, et al. Folate intake and colorectal cancer risk: a meta-analytical approach. Int J Cancer 2005;113:825-8.

Kennedy DA, Stern SJ, Moretti M, et al. Folate intake and the risk of colorectal cancer: a systematic review and meta-analysis. Cancer Epidemiol 2011;35:2-10.

Bassett JK, Severi G, Hodge AM, et al. Dietary intake of B vitamins and methionine and colorectal cancer risk. Nutr Cancer 2013;65:659-67.

de Vogel S, Dindore V, van Engeland M, et al. Dietary folate, methionine, riboflavin, and vitamin B-6 and risk of sporadic colorectal cancer. J Nutr 2008;138:2372-8.

Neuhouser ML, Cheng TY, Beresford SA, et al. Red blood cell folate and plasma folate are not associated with risk of incident colorectal cancer in the Women's Health Initiative observational study. Int J Cancer 2015;137:930-9.

Chuang SC, Rota M, Gunter MJ, et al. Quantifying the dose-response relationship between circulating folate concentrations and colorectal cancer in cohort studies: a meta-analysis based on a flexible meta-regression model. Am J Epidemiol 2013;178:1028-37.

Song Y, Manson JE, Lee IM, et al. Effect of combined folic acid, vitamin B(6), and vitamin B(12) on colorectal adenoma. J Natl Cancer Inst 2012;104:1562-75.

Figueiredo JC, Mott LA, Giovannucci E, et al. Folic acid and prevention of colorectal adenomas: a combined analysis of randomized clinical trials. Int J Cancer 2011;129:192-203.

De-Regil LM, Fernández-Gaxiola AC, Dowswell T, Peña-Rosas JP. Effects and safety of periconceptional folate supplementation for preventing birth defects. Cochrane Database Syst Rev. 2010 Oct 6;(10):CD007950. doi: 10.1002/14651858.CD007950.pub2. Update in: Cochrane Database Syst Rev. 2015;12:CD007950. PMID: 20927767; PMCID: PMC4160020.

Chapter 7 - Pre and Post Natal

Gernand AD, Schulze KJ, Stewart CP, West KP Jr, Christian P. Micronutrient deficiencies in pregnancy worldwide: health effects and prevention. Nat Rev Endocrinol. 2016 May;12(5):274-89. doi: 10.1038/nrendo.2016.37. Epub 2016 Apr 1. PMID: 27032981; PMCID: PMC4927329.

Centres for Disease Control and Prevention

Soma-Pillay P, Nelson-Piercy C, Tolppanen H, Mebazaa A. Physiological changes in pregnancy. Cardiovasc J Afr. 2016 Mar-Apr;27(2):89-94. doi: 10.5830/CVJA-2016-021. PMID: 27213856; PMCID: PMC4928162.

Makrides M, Gibson RA, McPhee AJ, Yelland L, Quinlivan J, Ryan P; DOMInO Investigative Team. Effect of DHA supplementation during pregnancy on maternal depression and neurodevelopment of young children: a randomized controlled trial. JAMA. 2010 Oct 20;304(15):1675-83. doi: 10.1001/jama.2010.1507. PMID: 20959577.

Elias J, Bozzo P, Einarson A. Are probiotics safe for use during pregnancy and lactation? Can Fam Physician. 2011 Mar;57(3):299-301. PMID: 21402964; PMCID: PMC3056676.

National Qualification in Pre and Post Natal Exercise - NTC

Caudill MA, Strupp BJ, Muscalu L, Nevins JEH, Canfield RL. Maternal choline supplementation during the third trimester of pregnancy improves infant information processing speed: a randomized, double-blind, controlled feeding study. FASEB J. 2018 Apr;32(4):2172-2180. doi: 10.1096/fj.201700692RR. Epub 2018 Jan 5. PMID: 29217669; PMCID: PMC6988845.

Chapter 8 - Perimenopause and Menopause

Lara briden - the hormone repair manual

Cleveland Clinic

Aguiar AF, Januário RS, Junior RP, Gerage AM, Pina FL, do Nascimento MA, Padovani CR, Cyrino ES. Long-term creatine supplementation improves muscular performance during resistance training in older women. Eur J Appl Physiol. 2013 Apr;113(4):987-96. doi: 10.1007/s00421-012-2514-6. Epub 2012 Oct 7. PMID: 23053133.

Kious BM, Kondo DG, Renshaw PF. Creatine for the Treatment of Depression. Biomolecules. 2019 Aug 23;9(9):406. doi: 10.3390/biom9090406. PMID: 31450809; PMCID: PMC6769464.

Examine.com

Allen MJ, Sharma S. Magnesium. [Updated 2021 Jul 25]. Treasure Island (FL): StatPearls Publishing; 2021 Jan-.

U.S. DEPARTMENT OF AGRICULTURE- https://fdc.nal.usda.gov/ndb/nutrients/index

Ciappolino V, Mazzocchi A, Enrico P, Syrén ML, Delvecchio G, Agostoni C, Brambilla P. N-3 Polyunsatured Fatty Acids in Menopausal Transition: A Systematic Review of Depressive and Cognitive Disorders with Accompanying Vasomotor Symptoms. Int J Mol Sci. 2018 Jun 23;19(7):1849. doi: 10.3390/ijms19071849. PMID: 29937484; PMCID: PMC6073395.

Patade A, Devareddy L, Lucas EA, Korlagunta K, Daggy BP, Arjmandi BH. Flaxseed reduces total and

LDL cholesterol concentrations in Native American postmenopausal women. J Womens Health (Larchmt). 2008 Apr;17(3):355-66. doi: 10.1089/jwh.2007.0359. PMID: 18328014.

van Die MD, Burger HG, Teede HJ, Bone KM. Vitex agnus-castus (Chaste-Tree/Berry) in the treatment of menopause-related complaints. J Altern Complement Med. 2009 Aug;15(8):853-62. doi: 10.1089/acm.2008.0447. PMID: 19678775.

van Die MD, Burger HG, Bone KM, Cohen MM, Teede HJ. Hypericum perforatum with Vitex agnus-castus in menopausal symptoms: a randomized, controlled trial. Menopause. 2009 Jan-Feb;16(1):156-63. doi: 10.1097/gme.0b013e31817fa9e0. PMID: 18791483.

Chopin Lucks B. Vitex agnus castus essential oil and menopausal balance: a research update [Complementary Therapies in Nursing and Midwifery 8 (2003) 148-154]. Complement Ther Nurs Midwifery. 2003 Aug;9(3):157-60. doi: 10.1016/S1353-6117(03)00020-9. PMID: 12852933.

Rizzoli R. Dairy products, yogurts, and bone health. Am J Clin Nutr. 2014 May;99(5 Suppl):1256S-62S. doi: 10.3945/ajcn.113.073056. Epub 2014 Apr 2. PMID: 24695889.

Durosier-Izart C, Biver E, Merminod F, van Rietbergen B, Chevalley T, Herrmann FR, Ferrari SL, Rizzoli R. Peripheral skeleton bone strength is positively correlated with total and dairy protein intakes in healthy postmenopausal women. Am J Clin Nutr. 2017 Feb;105(2):513-525. doi: 10.3945/ajcn.116.134676. Epub 2017 Jan 11. PMID: 28077378.

Parazzini F. Resveratrol, tryptophanum, glycine and vitamin E: a nutraceutical approach to sleep disturbance and irritability in peri- and post-menopause. Minerva Ginecol. 2015 Feb;67(1):1-5. PMID: 25660429.

Purdue-Smithe AC, Whitcomb BW, Szegda KL, Boutot ME, Manson JE, Hankinson SE, Rosner BA, Troy LM, Michels KB, Bertone-Johnson ER. Vitamin D and calcium intake and risk of early menopause. Am J Clin Nutr. 2017 Jun;105(6):1493-1501. doi: 10.3945/ajcn.116.145607. Epub 2017 May 10. PMID: 28490509; PMCID: PMC5445672.

Alkhalaf Z, Kim K, Kuhr DL, Radoc JG, Purdue-Smithe A, Pollack AZ, Yisahak SF, Silver RM, Thoma M, Kissell K, Perkins NJ, Sjaarda LA, Mumford SL. Markers of vitamin D metabolism and premenstrual symptoms in healthy women with regular cycles. Hum Reprod. 2021 Jun 18;36(7):1808-1820. doi: 10.1093/humrep/deab089. PMID: 33864070; PMCID: PMC8530167.

Aune D, Keum N, Giovannucci E, Fadnes LT, Boffetta P, Greenwood DC, Tonstad S, Vatten LJ, Riboli E, Norat T. Whole grain consumption and risk of cardiovascular disease, cancer, and all cause and cause specific mortality: systematic review and dose-response meta-analysis of prospective studies. BMJ. 2016 Jun 14;353:i2716. doi:

10.1136/bmj.i2716. PMID: 27301975; PMCID: PMC4908315.

Gil A, Ortega RM, Maldonado J. Wholegrain cereals and bread: a duet of the Mediterranean diet for the prevention of chronic diseases. Public Health Nutr. 2011 Dec;14(12A):2316-22. doi: 10.1017/S1368980011002576. PMID: 22166190.

Jacobs DR, Pereira MA, Meyer KA, Kushi LH. Fiber from whole grains, but not refined grains, is inversely associated with all-cause mortality in older women: the Iowa women's health study. J Am Coll Nutr. 2000 Jun;19(3 Suppl):326S-330S. doi: 10.1080/07315724.2000.10718968. PMID: 10875605.

Slavin JL, Lloyd B. Health benefits of fruits and vegetables. Adv Nutr. 2012 Jul 1;3(4):506-16. doi: 10.3945/an.112.002154. PMID: 22797986; PMCID: PMC3649719.

Kroenke CH, Caan BJ, Stefanick ML, Anderson G, Brzyski R, Johnson KC, LeBlanc E, Lee C, La Croix AZ, Park HL, Sims ST, Vitolins M, Wallace R. Effects of a dietary intervention and weight change on vasomotor symptoms in the Women's Health Initiative. Menopause. 2012 Sep;19(9):980-8. doi: 10.1097/gme.0b013e31824f606e. PMID: 22781782; PMCID: PMC3428489.

Fowke JH, Longcope C, Hebert JR. Brassica vegetable consumption shifts estrogen metabolism in healthy postmenopausal women. Cancer Epidemiol Biomarkers Prev. 2000 Aug;9(8):773-9.

PMID: 10952093.

Feresin RG, Johnson SA, Pourafshar S, Campbell JC, Jaime SJ, Navaei N, Elam ML, Akhavan NS, Alvarez-Alvarado S, Tenenbaum G, Brummel-Smith K, Salazar G, Figueroa A, Arjmandi BH. Impact of daily strawberry consumption on blood pressure and arterial stiffness in pre- and stage 1-hypertensive postmenopausal women: a randomized controlled trial. Food Funct. 2017 Nov 15;8(11):4139-4149. doi: 10.1039/c7fo01183k. PMID: 29099521.

Terauchi M, Horiguchi N, Kajiyama A, Akiyoshi M, Owa Y, Kato K, Kubota T. Effects of grape seed proanthocyanidin extract on menopausal symptoms, body composition, and cardiovascular parameters in middle-aged women: a randomized, double-blind, placebo-controlled pilot study. Menopause. 2014 Sep;21(9):990-6. doi: 10.1097/GME.0000000000000200. PMID: 24518152.

Bacciottini L, Falchetti A, Pampaloni B, Bartolini E, Carossino AM, Brandi ML. Phytoestrogens: food or drug? Clin Cases Miner Bone Metab. 2007 May;4(2):123-30. PMID: 22461212; PMCID: PMC2781234.

Bacciottini L, Falchetti A, Pampaloni B, Bartolini E, Carossino AM, Brandi ML. Phytoestrogens: food or drug? Clin Cases Miner Bone Metab. 2007 May;4(2):123-30. PMID: 22461212; PMCID: PMC2781234.

Hooper L, Ryder JJ, Kurzer MS, Lampe JW,

Messina MJ, Phipps WR, Cassidy A. Effects of soy protein and isoflavones on circulating hormone concentrations in pre- and post-menopausal women: a systematic review and meta-analysis. Hum Reprod Update. 2009 Jul-Aug;15(4):423-40. doi: 10.1093/humupd/dmp010. Epub 2009 Mar 19. PMID: 19299447; PMCID: PMC2691652.

Chen MN, Lin CC, Liu CF. Efficacy of phytoestrogens for menopausal symptoms: a meta-analysis and systematic review. Climacteric. 2015 Apr;18(2):260-9. doi: 10.3109/13697137.2014.966241. Epub 2014 Dec 1. PMID: 25263312; PMCID: PMC4389700.

Maltais ML, Desroches J, Dionne IJ. Changes in muscle mass and strength after menopause. J Musculoskelet Neuronal Interact. 2009 Oct-Dec;9(4):186-97. PMID: 19949277.

Rizzoli R, Stevenson JC, Bauer JM, van Loon LJ, Walrand S, Kanis JA, Cooper C, Brandi ML, Diez-Perez A, Reginster JY; ESCEO Task Force. The role of dietary protein and vitamin D in maintaining musculoskeletal health in postmenopausal women: a consensus statement from the European Society for Clinical and Economic Aspects of Osteoporosis and Osteoarthritis (ESCEO). Maturitas. 2014 Sep;79(1):122-32. doi: 10.1016/j.maturitas.2014.07.005. Epub 2014 Jul 17. Erratum in: Maturitas. 2015 Mar;80(3):337. PMID: 25082206.

König D, Oesser S, Scharla S, Zdzieblik D, Gollhofer A. Specific Collagen Peptides Improve Bone Mineral

Density and Bone Markers in Postmenopausal Women-A Randomized Controlled Study. Nutrients. 2018 Jan 16;10(1):97. doi: 10.3390/nu10010097. PMID: 29337906; PMCID: PMC5793325.

Fung TT, Meyer HE, Willett WC, Feskanich D. Protein intake and risk of hip fractures in postmenopausal women and men age 50 and older. Osteoporos Int. 2017 Apr;28(4):1401-1411. doi: 10.1007/s00198-016-3898-7. Epub 2017 Jan 10. PMID: 28074249; PMCID: PMC5357457.

Cagnacci A, Cannoletta M, Palma F, Zanin R, Xholli A, Volpe A. Menopausal symptoms and risk factors for cardiovascular disease in postmenopause. Climacteric. 2012 Apr;15(2):157-62. doi: 10.3109/13697137.2011.617852. Epub 2011 Dec 5. PMID: 22141325.

Thurston RC, El Khoudary SR, Sutton-Tyrrell K, Crandall CJ, Sternfeld B, Joffe H, Gold EB, Selzer F, Matthews KA. Vasomotor symptoms and insulin resistance in the study of women's health across the nation. J Clin Endocrinol Metab. 2012 Oct;97(10):3487-94. doi: 10.1210/jc.2012-1410. Epub 2012 Jul 31. PMID: 22851488; PMCID: PMC3462945.

Lee SW, Jo HH, Kim MR, Kwon DJ, You YO, Kim JH. Association between menopausal symptoms and metabolic syndrome in postmenopausal women. Arch Gynecol Obstet. 2012 Feb;285(2):541-8. doi: 10.1007/s00404-011-2016-5. Epub 2011 Aug 19. PMID: 21853251.

Fardet A. Minimally processed foods are more satiating and less hyperglycemic than ultra-processed foods: a preliminary study with 98 ready-to-eat foods. Food Funct. 2016 May 18;7(5):2338-46. doi: 10.1039/c6fo00107f. Epub 2016 Apr 29. PMID: 27125637.

Archer DF, Sturdee DW, Baber R, de Villiers TJ, Pines A, Freedman RR, Gompel A, Hickey M, Hunter MS, Lobo RA, Lumsden MA, MacLennan AH, Maki P, Palacios S, Shah D, Villaseca P, Warren M. Menopausal hot flushes and night sweats: where are we now? Climacteric. 2011 Oct;14(5):515-28. doi: 10.3109/13697137.2011.608596. Epub 2011 Aug 18. PMID: 21848495.

Faubion SS, Sood R, Thielen JM, Shuster LT. Caffeine and menopausal symptoms: what is the association? Menopause. 2015 Feb;22(2):155-8. doi: 10.1097/GME.0000000000000301. PMID: 25051286.

Pimenta F, Leal I, Maroco J, Ramos C. Perceived control, lifestyle, health, socio-demographic factors and menopause: impact on hot flashes and night sweats. Maturitas. 2011 Aug;69(4):338-42. doi: 10.1016/j.maturitas.2011.05.005. Epub 2011 Jun 15. PMID: 21680119.

Hunter MS, Gupta P, Chedraui P, Blümel JE, Tserotas K, Aguirre W, Palacios S, Sturdee DW. The International Menopause Study of Climate, Altitude, Temperature (IMS-CAT) and vasomotor symptoms. Climacteric. 2013 Feb;16(1):8-16. doi: 10.3109/13697137.2012.699563. Epub 2012 Sep 4.

PMID: 22946508.

Stefanopoulou E, Shah D, Shah R, Gupta P, Sturdee DW, Hunter MS. An International Menopause Society study of climate, altitude, temperature (IMS-CAT) and vasomotor symptoms in urban Indian regions. Climacteric. 2014 Aug;17(4):417-24. doi: 10.3109/13697137.2013.852169. Epub 2013 Nov 7. PMID: 24099134.

Kwon SJ, Ha YC, Park Y. High dietary sodium intake is associated with low bone mass in postmenopausal women: Korea National Health and Nutrition Examination Survey, 2008-2011. Osteoporos Int. 2017 Apr;28(4):1445-1452. doi: 10.1007/s00198-017-3904-8. Epub 2017 Jan 10. PMID: 28074252.

Hernandez Schulman I, Raij L. Salt sensitivity and hypertension after menopause: role of nitric oxide and angiotensin II. Am J Nephrol. 2006;26(2):170-80. doi: 10.1159/000092984. Epub 2006 Apr 25. PMID: 16645264.

Torres SJ, Nowson CA. A moderate-sodium DASH-type diet improves mood in postmenopausal women. Nutrition. 2012 Sep;28(9):896-900. doi: 10.1016/j.nut.2011.11.029. Epub 2012 Apr 4. PMID: 22480799.

Lovejoy JC. The influence of sex hormones on obesity across the female life span. J Womens Health. 1998 Dec;7(10):1247-56. doi: 10.1089/jwh.1998.7.1247. PMID: 9929857.

Wing RR, Matthews KA, Kuller LH, Meilahn EN, Plantinga PL. Weight gain at the time of menopause. Arch Intern Med. 1991 Jan;151(1):97-102. PMID: 1985614.

Sowers M, Zheng H, Tomey K, Karvonen-Gutierrez C, Jannausch M, Li X, Yosef M, Symons J. Changes in body composition in women over six years at midlife: ovarian and chronological aging. J Clin Endocrinol Metab. 2007 Mar;92(3):895-901. doi: 10.1210/jc.2006-1393. Epub 2006 Dec 27. PMID: 17192296; PMCID: PMC2714766.

Sowers MR, Wildman RP, Mancuso P, Eyvazzadeh AD, Karvonen-Gutierrez CA, Rillamas-Sun E, Jannausch ML. Change in adipocytokines and ghrelin with menopause. Maturitas. 2008 Feb 20;59(2):149-57. doi: 10.1016/j.maturitas.2007.12.006. Epub 2008 Feb 14. PMID: 18280066; PMCID: PMC2311418.

Boonyaratanakornkit V, Pateetin P. The role of ovarian sex steroids in metabolic homeostasis, obesity, and postmenopausal breast cancer: molecular mechanisms and therapeutic implications. Biomed Res Int. 2015;2015:140196. doi: 10.1155/2015/140196. Epub 2015 Mar 19. PMID: 25866757; PMCID: PMC4383469.

https://www.ncbi.nlm.nih.gov/pmc/articles/PMC3964739/

Zsakai A, Karkus Z, Utczas K, Biri B, Sievert LL, Bodzsar EB. Body fatness and endogenous sex hormones in the menopausal transition. Maturitas. 2016 May;87:18-26. doi: 10.1016/j.maturitas.2016.02.006. Epub 2016 Feb 12. PMID: 27013284.

Messier V, Rabasa-Lhoret R, Barbat-Artigas S, Elisha B, Karelis AD, Aubertin-Leheudre M. Menopause and sarcopenia: A potential role for sex hormones. Maturitas. 2011 Apr;68(4):331-6. doi: 10.1016/j.maturitas.2011.01.014. Epub 2011 Feb 25. PMID: 21353405.

Proudler AJ, Felton CV, Stevenson JC. Ageing and the response of plasma insulin, glucose and C-peptide concentrations to intravenous glucose in postmenopausal women. Clin Sci (Lond). 1992 Oct;83(4):489-94. doi: 10.1042/cs0830489. PMID: 1330412.

Salpeter SR, Walsh JM, Ormiston TM, Greyber E, Buckley NS, Salpeter EE. Meta-analysis: effect of hormone-replacement therapy on components of the metabolic syndrome in postmenopausal women. Diabetes Obes Metab. 2006 Sep;8(5):538-54. doi: 10.1111/j.1463-1326.2005.00545.x. PMID: 16918589.

Gower BA, Goss AM. A lower-carbohydrate, higher-fat diet reduces abdominal and intermuscular fat and increases insulin sensitivity in adults at risk of type 2 diabetes. J Nutr. 2015 Jan;145(1):177S-83S. doi: 10.3945/jn.114.195065. Epub 2014 Dec 3. PMID: 25527677; PMCID: PMC4264021.

Volek JS, Feinman RD. Carbohydrate restriction

improves the features of Metabolic Syndrome. Metabolic Syndrome may be defined by the response to carbohydrate restriction. Nutr Metab (Lond). 2005 Nov 16;2:31. doi: 10.1186/1743-7075-2-31. PMID: 16288655; PMCID: PMC1323303.

Brahe LK, Le Chatelier E, Prifti E, Pons N, Kennedy S, Blædel T, Håkansson J, Dalsgaard TK, Hansen T, Pedersen O, Astrup A, Ehrlich SD, Larsen LH. Dietary modulation of the gut microbiota--a randomised controlled trial in obese postmenopausal women. Br J Nutr. 2015 Aug 14;114(3):406-17. doi: 10.1017/S0007114515001786. Epub 2015 Jul 2. PMID: 26134388; PMCID: PMC4531470.

Conceição MS, Bonganha V, Vechin FC, Berton RP, Lixandrão ME, Nogueira FR, de Souza GV, Chacon-Mikahil MP, Libardi CA. Sixteen weeks of resistance training can decrease the risk of metabolic syndrome in healthy postmenopausal women. Clin Interv Aging. 2013;8:1221-8. doi: 10.2147/CIA.S44245. Epub 2013 Sep 16. PMID: 24072967; PMCID: PMC3783540.

Thiebaud RS, Loenneke JP, Fahs CA, Rossow LM, Kim D, Abe T, Anderson MA, Young KC, Bemben DA, Bemben MG. The effects of elastic band resistance training combined with blood flow restriction on strength, total bone-free lean body mass and muscle thickness in postmenopausal women. Clin Physiol Funct Imaging. 2013 Sep;33(5):344-52. doi: 10.1111/cpf.12033. Epub 2013 Apr 3. PMID: 23701116.

Nedeltcheva AV, Scheer FA. Metabolic effects of

sleep disruption, links to obesity and diabetes. Curr Opin Endocrinol Diabetes Obes. 2014 Aug;21(4):293-8. doi: 10.1097/MED.0000000000000082. PMID: 24937041; PMCID: PMC4370346.

NHS

Faubion SS, Sood R, Thielen JM, Shuster LT. Caffeine and menopausal symptoms: what is the association? Menopause. 2015 Feb;22(2):155-8. doi: 10.1097/GME.0000000000000301. PMID: 25051286.

Pimenta F, Leal I, Maroco J, Ramos C. Perceived control, lifestyle, health, socio-demographic factors and menopause: impact on hot flashes and night sweats. Maturitas. 2011 Aug;69(4):338-42. doi: 10.1016/j.maturitas.2011.05.005. Epub 2011 Jun 15. PMID: 21680119.

Mograbi GJ. Meditation and the brain: attention, control and emotion. Mens Sana Monogr. 2011 Jan;9(1):276-83. doi: 10.4103/0973-1229.77444. PMID: 21694979; PMCID: PMC3115297.

Maki PM, Henderson VW. Cognition and the menopause transition. Menopause. 2016 Jul;23(7):803-5. doi: 10.1097/GME.0000000000000681. PMID: 27272226.

Weber MT, Rubin LH, Maki PM. Cognition in perimenopause: the effect of transition stage. Menopause. 2013 May;20(5):511-7. doi:

10.1097/gme.0b013e31827655e5. PMID: 23615642; PMCID: PMC3620712.

Sleep Foundation

Weber MT, Rubin LH, Maki PM. Cognition in perimenopause: the effect of transition stage. Menopause. 2013 May;20(5):511-7. doi: 10.1097/gme.0b013e31827655e5. PMID: 23615642; PMCID: PMC3620712.

Chiu HY, Yeh TH, Huang YC, Chen PY. Effects of Intravenous and Oral Magnesium on Reducing Migraine: A Meta-analysis of Randomized Controlled Trials. Pain Physician. 2016 Jan;19(1):E97-112. PMID: 26752497.

Boehnke C, Reuter U, Flach U, Schuh-Hofer S, Einhäupl KM, Arnold G. High-dose riboflavin treatment is efficacious in migraine prophylaxis: an open study in a tertiary care centre. Eur J Neurol. 2004 Jul;11(7):475-7. doi: 10.1111/j.1468-1331.2004.00813.x. PMID: 15257686.

Chapter 9 - Thyroid

National Institute of Diabetes and Digestive and Kidney issues
https://www.niddk.nih.gov/health-information/endocrine-diseases/hypothyroidism

Thanh D. Hoang, Cara H. Olsen, Vinh Q. Mai, Patrick W. Clyde, Mohamed K. M. Shakir, Desiccated Thyroid Extract Compared With

Levothyroxine in the Treatment of Hypothyroidism: A Randomized, Double-Blind, Crossover Study, The Journal of Clinical Endocrinology & Metabolism, Volume 98, Issue 5, 1 May 2013, Pages 1982–1990, https://doi.org/10.1210/jc.2012-4107

Franklyn JA, Boelaert K. Thyrotoxicosis. Lancet. 2012 Mar 24;379(9821):1155-66. doi: 10.1016/S0140-6736(11)60782-4. Epub 2012 Mar 5. PMID: 22394559.

Bathla M, Singh M, Relan P. Prevalence of anxiety and depressive symptoms among patients with hypothyroidism. Indian J Endocrinol Metab. 2016 Jul-Aug;20(4):468-74. doi: 10.4103/2230-8210.183476. PMID: 27366712; PMCID: PMC4911835.

NHS - https://www.nhs.uk/conditions/overactive-thyroid-hyperthyroidism/treatment/

Badawy A, State O, Sherief S. Can thyroid dysfunction explicate severe menopausal symptoms? J Obstet Gynaecol. 2007 Jul;27(5):503-5. doi: 10.1080/01443610701405812. PMID: 17701801.

Biondi B, Klein I. Hypothyroidism as a risk factor for cardiovascular disease. Endocrine. 2004 Jun;24(1):1-13. doi: 10.1385/ENDO:24:1:001. PMID: 15249698.

Chapter 10 - Your cycle leaves Clues

Morgan A. Pratte, Kaushal B. Nanavati, Virginia Young, and Christopher P. Morley.The Journal of Alternative and Complementary Medicine.Dec 2014.901-908.http://doi.org/10.1089/acm.2014.0177

Navvabi Rigi, S., kermansaravi, F., Navidian, A. et al. Comparing the analgesic effect of heat patch containing iron chip and ibuprofen for primary dysmenorrhea: a randomized controlled trial. BMC Women's Health 12, 25 (2012). https://doi.org/10.1186/1472-6874-12-25

Valiani M, Ghasemi N, Bahadoran P, Heshmat R. The effects of massage therapy on dysmenorrhea caused by endometriosis. Iran J Nurs Midwifery Res. 2010 Fall;15(4):167-71. PMID: 21589790; PMCID: PMC3093183.

Whipple B, Komisaruk BR. Elevation of pain threshold by vaginal stimulation in women. Pain. 1985 Apr;21(4):357-367. doi: 10.1016/0304-3959(85)90164-2. PMID: 4000685.

Srivastava JK, Shankar E, Gupta S. Chamomile: A herbal medicine of the past with a bright future. Mol Med Rep. 2010 Nov 1;3(6):895-901. doi: 10.3892/mmr.2010.377. PMID: 21132119; PMCID: PMC2995283.

Giti Ozgoli, Marjan Goli, and Fariborz Moattar.The Journal of Alternative and Complementary Medicine.Feb 2009.129-132.http://doi.org/10.1089/acm.2008.0311

Heidarifar R, Mehran N, Heidari A, Tehran HA,

Koohbor M, Mansourabad MK. Effect of Dill (Anethum graveolens) on the severity of primary dysmenorrhea in compared with mefenamic acid: A randomized, double-blind trial. J Res Med Sci. 2014 Apr;19(4):326-30. PMID: 25097605; PMCID: PMC4115348.

Seifert B, Wagler P, Dartsch S, Schmidt U, Nieder J. Magnesium--eine therapeutische Alternative bei der primären Dysmenorrhoe [Magnesium--a new therapeutic alternative in primary dysmenorrhea]. Zentralbl Gynakol. 1989;111(11):755-60. German. PMID: 2675496.

Eby GA. Zinc treatment prevents dysmenorrhea. Med Hypotheses. 2007;69(2):297-301. doi: 10.1016/j.mehy.2006.12.009. Epub 2007 Feb 7. PMID: 17289285.

Zekavat OR, Karimi MY, Amanat A, Alipour F. A randomised controlled trial of oral zinc sulphate for primary dysmenorrhoea in adolescent females. Aust N Z J Obstet Gynaecol. 2015 Aug;55(4):369-73. doi: 10.1111/ajo.12367. Epub 2015 Jun 30. PMID: 26132140.

Nagma S, Kapoor G, Bharti R, Batra A, Batra A, Aggarwal A, Sablok A. To evaluate the effect of perceived stress on menstrual function. J Clin Diagn Res. 2015 Mar;9(3):QC01-3. doi: 10.7860/JCDR/2015/6906.5611. Epub 2015 Mar 1. PMID: 25954667; PMCID: PMC4413117.

Villavicencio J, Allen RH. Unscheduled bleeding and contraceptive choice: increasing satisfaction and continuation rates. Open Access J Contracept. 2016 Mar 31;7:43-52. doi: 10.2147/OAJC.S85565. PMID: 29386936; PMCID: PMC5683158.

Fraser IS, Mansour D, Breymann C, Hoffman C, Mezzacasa A, Petraglia F. Prevalence of heavy menstrual bleeding and experiences of affected women in a European patient survey. Int J Gynaecol Obstet. 2015 Mar;128(3):196–200.

Melmed, S., & Williams, R. H. (2011). Williams textbook of endocrinology (12th ed.). Philadelphia: Elsevier/Saunders. Page 68.

Poppe K, Velkeniers B, Glinoer D. Thyroid disease and female reproduction. Clin Endocrinol (Oxf). 2007 Mar;66(3):309–21.

Squizzato A, Romualdi E, Büller HR, Gerdes VE. Clinical review: Thyroid dysfunction and effects on coagulation and fibrinolysis: a systematic review. J Clin Endocrinol Metab. 2007 Jul;92(7):2415–20.

Stoffer SS. Menstrual disorders and mild thyroid insufficiency: intriguing cases suggesting an association. Postgrad Med. 1982 Aug;72(2):75–7, 80–2.

NHS - https://www.nhs.uk/conditions/heavy-periods/treatment/

Livdans-Forret AB, Harvey PJ, Larkin-Thier SM. Menorrhagia: a synopsis of management focusing on herbal and nutritional supplements, and chiropractic. J Can Chiropr Assoc. 2007

Dec;51(4):235-46. PMID: 18060009; PMCID: PMC2077876.

Marshall LM, Spiegelman D, Goldman MB, Manson JE, Colditz GA, Barbieri RL, Stampfer MJ, Hunter DJ. A prospective study of reproductive factors and oral contraceptive use in relation to the risk of uterine leiomyomata. Fertil Steril. 1998 Sep;70(3):432-9. doi: 10.1016/s0015-0282(98)00208-8. PMID: 9757871.

Mayo Clinic

NHS

Dalton-Brewer, N. The Role of Complementary and Alternative Medicine for the Management of Fibroids and Associated Symptomatology. Curr Obstet Gynecol Rep 5, 110–118 (2016). https://doi.org/10.1007/s13669-016-0156-0

Baird DD, Hill MC, Schectman JM, Hollis BW. Vitamin d and the risk of uterine fibroids. Epidemiology. 2013 May;24(3):447-53. doi: 10.1097/EDE.0b013e31828acca0. PMID: 23493030; PMCID: PMC5330388.

Printed in Great Britain
by Amazon